A Practical Guide to Managing Paediatric Problems on the Postnatal Wards

A Practical Guide to Managing Paediatric Problems on the Postnatal Wards

Edited by

CHRISTOPHER FLANNIGAN

Radcliffe Publishing
Oxford • New York

Radcliffe Publishing Ltd
18 Marcham Road
Abingdon
Oxon OX14 1AA
United Kingdom

www.radcliffepublishing.com
Electronic catalogue and worldwide online ordering facility.

British Library Cataloguing in Publication Data

A catalogue record for this book is available from the British Library.

ISBN-13: 978 1 84619 506 8

The paper used for the text pages of this book
is FSC certified. FSC® (The Forest Stewardship
Council®) is an international network to promote
responsible management of the world's forests.

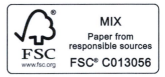

MIX
Paper from
responsible sources
FSC® C013056

Typeset by Pindar NZ, Auckland, New Zealand
Printed and bound by TJI Digital, Padstow, Cornwall, UK

Contents

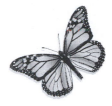

Foreword	vii
About the editor	ix
About the contributors	x
Acknowledgements	xi

1 The newborn check	**1**
2 Examination abnormalities	**7**
Scalp swelling	7
Abnormal red reflex	11
Preauricular skin tags	14
Facial nerve palsy	15
Tongue-tie	16
Cleft lip and palate	18
Fractured clavicle	20
Erb's palsy	21
Single palmar crease	22
Breast swelling	23
Heart murmurs	24
Absent femorals	26
Abnormal hips	28
Two-cord vessels	30
Umbilical hernia	32
Divarication of the recti	33
Inguinal hernia	34
Undescended testes	35
Hydroceles	37
Hypospadias	39
Talipes	41
Sacral dimple	43

Bruising 45

Birthmarks 47

Rashes 49

3 Clinical problems 51

Respiratory distress 51

Cyanosis 54

Tachycardia 56

Bradycardia 58

Sepsis 59

Jaundice 64

Hypoglycaemia 70

Poor feeding 77

Weight loss >10% 80

Vomiting 82

Jittery 84

Not passed urine 86

Bowels not opened 88

Sticky eyes 89

Redness around umbilical cord 91

Pink staining on nappy 93

Vaginal bleeding 94

Maternal thyroid disease 95

Maternal hepatitis B 97

BCG vaccination 99

Vitamin K 101

Notes 103

Further reading 107

DVD contents 108

Index 109

Foreword

Why buy this book?

If you're a young doctor, midwife or other professional commencing a post involving the care of normal newborn babies, take interest.

This book has been developed as an 'A–Z' of most of the clinical problems you will face – with answers as to what to do, how to counsel parents, and how to manage all of the common scenarios. You may already be worrying about your rotation or have started your post and feel out of your depth: this book is designed to take away the 'mystery' of newborn transition and provide easy access to all the background information you will need, with practical solutions.

Hence, if you need to understand the reasons behind the 'newborn examination', if you're not sure what to do if you hear a murmur in a baby, what the features of 'sepsis' might be or how to go about managing jaundice, you will find the answers here. We know that newborn babies are different from any of the 'patients' you will have encountered before – even the amount of milk or fluid a baby requires necessitates a calculation – and this book is designed to help explain the common issues and make things easy for those involved in their care, from the start.

We have sought to produce a user-friendly resource, whilst additionally ensured extensive references are included for those wishing to read further. Themed subheadings covering background information, clinical history and examination, and management are used for all topics. Some of the most important issues, which merit early consideration by postnatal staff, are the subject of audio-visual slideshow presentations contained in the included DVD. The presentations cover jaundice, hypoglycaemia, common problems related to the newborn examination and a discussion on the neonatal management of antenatally detected renal tract dilation.

The DVD is designed to compliment the book, and in addition includes a video demonstration of the newborn examination.

The authors include experienced consultant neonatologists and senior trainees who deal regularly with the recurrent themes of day-to-day newborn care, and are sensitive to the needs of younger trainees and staff who may feel 'isolated' with the charge of 'getting on with the job' in busy maternity units. We have been concerned that despite good intentions and efforts to supervise, all too often junior doctors and midwives find themselves 'in at the deep end' at the start of a 'postnatal' rotation and may struggle for weeks or months without adequate orientation or instruction.

If you are one of those professionals, we hope this book might go some way to 'close the knowledge gap' and provide the practical tools to assist you for the better care of your patients.

Dr Phil Quinn
Consultant Neonatologist and Paediatrician
Craigavon Area Hospital
November 2010

About the editor

Dr Christopher Flannigan MB BCh BAO DCH MRCPCH
Dr Christopher Flannigan is a paediatric registrar working in the Northern
Ireland Deanery. He has a special interest in electronic learning.

About the contributors

Dr Martina Hogan MB BCh BAO DCH D.Obs FRCPCH MBA
Dr Martina Hogan is a neonatologist and works at Craigavon Area Hospital. She has an interest in multidisciplinary working within the healthcare setting and quality improvement.
Contributions – The newborn check chapter and video

Dr Phil Quinn MB BCh BAO DCH MRCPCH FRACP
Dr Phil Quinn is a consultant neonatologist and paediatrician working in Craigavon Area Hospital. Dr Quinn trained in the UK and Melbourne, Australia. He has a special interest in newborn ventilatory support and teaching in neonatology and paediatrics.
Contributions – Foreword and audio presentations

Dr David Sweet MD FRCPCH
Dr David Sweet is a consultant neonatologist working in the Royal Maternity Hospital in Belfast.
Contributions – Heart murmurs

Dr Victor Morris MBBS MRCPCH
Dr Victor Morris is a paediatric registrar working in the Royal Maternity Hospital in Belfast.
Contributions – Hypospadias, Jaundice and Hypoglycaemia

Acknowledgements

This book is dedicated to my wife Michelle. I would like to thank Michelle for her patience and support while this book was being written.

I would also like to thank my father Stephen for his contribution to the electronic components of this package; without his hard work and expertise so much of this project would not have been possible.

I would like to thank Dr Richard Tubman and Dr David Grier for carrying out the peer review. Their contribution has added significantly to the finished product and their hard work is greatly appreciated.

Finally, I would like to thank Malcolm Battin from Newborn Services, Auckland City Hospital, Sue Carroll from the Cleft Lip & Palate Association (CLAPA), and Daniel J Hatch from the Foot & Ankle Center of Northern Colorado PC, for providing images for the book.

1. The newborn check

Introduction

➤ A considerable amount of information can be obtained prior to touching the infant. The newborn examination is a good screening test as early detection of abnormalities can allow treatment before an illness occurs.

➤ Talk with the midwife and the mother.

➤ Read the mother's notes and familiarise yourself with the hand-held records.

➤ Note the family and social history, mother's personal and reproductive history, this pregnancy, labour and delivery.

➤ Note the gestational age, duration of labour, presence of fetal heart rate anomalies, duration of second stage of labour, placental or amniotic fluid abnormalities. The normality scan report and mother's blood group should be noted.

➤ Note the baby's age and his/her feeding pattern.

➤ The examination should be carried out in the presence of the baby's mother.

General appearance

➤ Look at the baby; you will be able to assess the colour, posture, tone, activity maturity and quality of cry.

Cardiac examination

➤ Do this part of the newborn check first while the infant is quiet – usually at the beginning of the examination.

➤ Ensure you have washed your hands and wipe the stethoscope with a sterile wipe.

➤ Place the palm of your hand over the heart to locate the apex beat and note the presence of any heaves or thrills.

➤ Listen for heart sounds over the apex, lower left sternal edge, pulmonary area and aortic area and assess quality of heart sounds one and two. Listen for murmurs, noting the location and quality of the murmur.

➤ Assess heart rate (normally 120–160 beats per minute).

➤ Hold the infant's thighs and feel femoral pulses when the infant is quiet. The pulses should be equal and strong. Assess for radio-femoral delay by feeling the brachial and femoral pulses simultaneously.

➤ Listen for breath sounds and note the respiratory rate (normal rate 40–60 breaths per minute).

➤ Any abnormality will require investigation.

Head and neck

➤ Look at the shape of the head; there may be swelling or oedema. Gentle but firm palpation will help you distinguish between caput succedaneum and cephalhaematoma. A caput crosses the suture lines whereas a cephalhaematoma does not. There may be moulding and overriding sutures. Check the anterior and posterior fontanelles.

➤ Assess the ear shape and position, looking for preauricular tags. Assess the infant's ear position: the upper part of the ear should transect an arbitrary line drawn through the inter canthus of both eyes and extrapolated laterally in the horizontal plane. If the upper part of the ear does not reach this line, consider that the ears are low set or posteriorly rotated.

➤ Look for nasal flaring or respiratory distress. The palate should be examined to ensure there is no cleft present.

➤ Infants have short, fat necks. There should be full mobility of the neck from right to left. Check for fractured clavicles by placing steady pressure from the outer aspect of the clavicle at the shoulder over to sternum. Crepitus and a stand-off can be felt if a fracture is present.

Abdomen

➤ Palpate the abdomen gently. Assess for abdominal masses and palpate the kidneys.

➤ Check for the presence of three-cord vessels if the cord is still fresh.

➤ Check for anal patency.

➤ Ensure the infant has passed meconium and urine.

Genitalia

➤ In girls the labia majora and minora should be seen. A white mucoid discharge is normal.

➤ In boys the penile shaft should be straight with an intact foreskin. Testes should be palpable.

Hip examination

➤ Check for symmetry of the limbs and skin folds.

➤ Ortolani's manoeuvre attempts to relocate a dislocated hip. The hips are abducted with the hips and knees flexed. The thighs should be able to abduct until they are flat against the examination table.

The clunk represents the passive reduction of the femoral head back into the acetabulum.

➤ Barlow's manoeuvre attempts to dislocate a dislocatable hip. Gentle but firm pressure directly posteriorly on the proximal medial thigh by the thumb while the hip is adducted elicits a clunk with subluxation or dislocation of the hip.[1]

Feet

➤ Check for talipes equinovarus, where the foot points downwards at the ankle (equinus), the heel is turned in (varus), the mid-foot is deviated towards the midline (adductus) and the first metatarsal points downwards (plantar flexion).[2] This is the most common abnormality with an incidence of 1.2 per thousand live births. The deformity is not passively correctable by the examiner.

Neurological

➤ Observe tone, behaviour, movements and posture.

➤ Check for normal grasp and Moro startle reflex. It is not possible to elicit the Moro reflex in a crying infant.

Spine examination

➤ Inspect and palpate bony structures and check integrity of the skin.

➤ A 'simple dimple' is defined as a midline dimple measuring <5 mm, located within 2.5 cm of the anus and not associated with any other cutaneous findings.[3]

➤ Dimples associated with haemangiomas, cutis aplasia or raised lesions require investigation – ultrasound or MRI.[4]

Opthalmology

Check for eye symmetry and shape of the eyes. The red reflex can be seen through an ophthalmoscope. The infant's eyes will spontaneously open if he/she is held upright and not disturbed too much.

Documentation

➤ Document the weight, head circumference and length in the parent-held child record (the 'red book'). Attention to detail is important.

➤ This examination should only take a few minutes; the documentation is important and forms a baseline for subsequent examinations.

2. Examination abnormalities

Scalp swelling

This is a common finding, particularly after birth by instrumental delivery. There are a number of common types of scalp swelling you should be able to identify and differentiate from the uncommon, but potentially life-threatening subaponeurotic haemorrhage.

➤ **Caput succedaneum** – This is oedema of the scalp secondary to pressure on the head during the delivery process. The oedema can extend across the midline and crosses suture lines.

➤ **Chignon** – This is superficial swelling/bleeding on an infant's scalp related to the application of a ventouse suction device. The area of swelling is circular in the shape of the suction cap and can cross both the midline and the suture lines.

➤ **Cephalhaematoma** – This is bleeding between the periosteum and the skull. In view of its anatomical location it does not cross the suture lines. It is most commonly found over the parietal region.

➤ **Subaponeurotic (subgaleal) haemorrhage** – This potentially lethal scalp swelling occurs secondary to rupture of veins running between the scalp and the dural sinuses. The rupture of these blood vessels is often associated with a ventouse delivery. Bleeding occurs into the space between the aponeurosis of the scalp and the periosteum. As this space is large, the infant can lose most of its blood volume into the space, presenting with signs of hypovolaemic shock. The scalp swelling is soft and fluctuant. It is not restricted by suture lines and can involve all of the scalp, although in the early stages it may be confined to the occipital region.

History and examination

➤ Enquire about the delivery – was it difficult? Were forceps or a ventouse required? Has the infant had vitamin K?

➤ Examine the scalp and note the consistency of the swelling, its location and whether it crosses suture lines or the midline.

➤ Examine for bruising elsewhere.

➤ Make sure the infant has no associated injuries, e.g. facial nerve palsy from a forceps delivery or a fractured clavicle/Erb's palsy from a difficult delivery complicated by a shoulder dystocia.

➤ If a subaponeurotic haemorrhage is suspected, assess for signs of blood loss/hypovolaemic shock, e.g. pallor, drowsiness, tachycardia and prolonged capillary refill time. Measure the head circumference at birth and frequently thereafter.

Management

➤ The parents should be reassured that most scalp swelling should settle over the next few days to weeks. Caput succedaneum generally resolves before a chignon, which tends to resolve more quickly than a cephalhaematoma. In the case of cephalhaematoma the parents should be warned that it can calcify as it heals resulting in a residual swelling.

➤ Any scalp swelling involving bruising/bleeding increases the risk of the infant developing jaundice and there should be a low threshold for checking the serum bilirubin if the infant appears jaundiced.

➤ If the infant seems in pain from the scalp swelling, paracetamol can be prescribed, at an appropriate dose.

➤ If there is any concern regarding excessive or widespread bruising, make sure the infant received postnatal vitamin K and check a full blood picture and clotting screen.

➤ If there is any concern about a subaponeurotic haemorrhage, ask for a senior opinion at once. If the infant has signs of shock, begin fluid resuscitation and admit to the neonatal unit without delay.

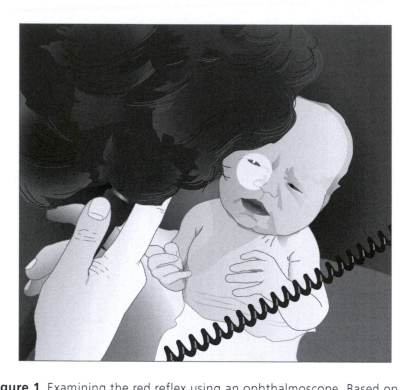

Figure 1 Examining the red reflex using an ophthalmoscope. Based on images courtesy of Newborn Services, Auckland City Hospital.

Abnormal red reflex

All babies should have both eyes examined for a red reflex as part of the routine neonatal discharge examination to detect conditions such as congenital cataracts or retinoblastoma.

History and examination

➤ Enquire about inherited eye disorders.

➤ Examine the red reflex in both eyes using an ophthalmoscope and compare for asymmetry.

➤ This is often one of the most difficult tasks on routine discharge examination as a newborn baby will often keep its eyes closed. Tips for examining the eyes include:

1   If the baby's eyes are open when you start the check, examine them first.

2   Keep your ophthalmoscope close to hand during the baby check so if the eyes open at any stage you will be ready.

3   If still not opening the eyes, manoeuvres to help include going to a dark area, getting the baby to suck, getting the mother to hold the baby and holding the baby vertically against the chest looking over the mother's shoulder.

4   If all these fail and the baby is relaxed you can gently try and open the eyes.

5   If you are unable to open the eyes you will have to try again at a later stage.

Management

➤ If there is a family history of inherited eye disease, major neurodevelopmental disorder, dysmorphic syndrome or abnormal red reflex, the baby should be referred to an ophthalmologist.

➤ There should be no delay in the referral, particularly if there is concern about an abnormal red reflex, as paediatric ophthalmologists advise that dense unilateral cataracts should be operated on within 6–8 weeks of birth and that bilateral cataracts are operated on between 3–6 months of age to ensure a good visual outcome and prevent amblyopia from developing.

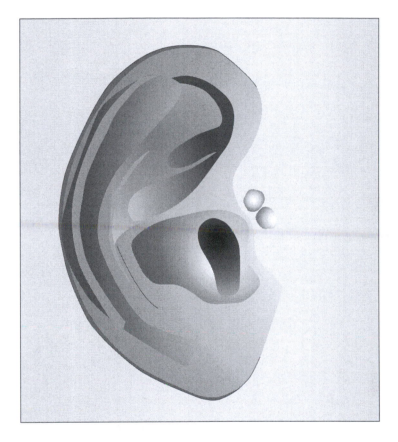

Figure 2 Preauricular skin tags. Based on images courtesy of Newborn Services, Auckland City Hospital.[6]

Preauricular skin tags

There is insufficient evidence to support the routine use of renal ultrasound in all infants with preauricular skin tags or pits. However, when other malformations or dysmorphic features are present, a renal ultrasound should be performed.[5]

History and examination

➤ Examine the infant for any dysmorphic features or malformations.

➤ Review the results of the infant's screening hearing tests.

Management

➤ Discuss the removal of the skin tags with the parents and offer routine outpatient referral to a plastic surgeon.

➤ If there are no dysmorphic features or other malformations, no further investigation is necessary.

➤ If there are dysmorphic features or other malformations present, organise a renal ultrasound and consult with your senior regarding further investigations.

Facial nerve palsy

Lower motor neuron facial nerve palsy occurs due to extrinsic compression on the facial nerve. It most commonly occurs during the delivery process as the infant's head is compressed against the mother's pelvis, but it can also be iatrogenic, e.g. after forceps delivery.

History and examination

➤ Inspect the face for asymmetry, which is most evident when the infant is crying. Here you will note that the mouth is pulled towards the normal side and there will be lack of wrinkling on the affected side.

➤ Document whether the infant is able to close the eye on the affected side.

➤ Look for evidence of a forceps mark or bruising over where the facial nerve emerges from the stylomastoid foramen.

➤ Ensure the rest of the nervous system examination is normal.

Management

➤ The mechanism of the facial nerve injury and the fact that most infants make a full recovery should be explained to the parents.

➤ If the infant is unable to close the eye, artificial tears should be prescribed.

➤ It is important to monitor feeding as the paralysis of the facial muscles can affect the infant's ability to latch on.

➤ Early outpatient follow-up should be arranged. If recovery is limited, further investigation may be required to exclude other causes of facial nerve palsy, e.g. Möbius syndrome, congenital absence of the facial muscles or intracranial haemorrhage.[7]

Tongue-tie

A tongue-tie is a relatively common condition found in about 1 in 20 babies. The frenulum under the tongue is short and appears to tether the tongue to the underside of the mouth. It usually does not cause any problems, but is often a major concern for the parents.

Management

➤ Reassurance for parents that an uncomplicated tongue-tie does not require any treatment.

➤ If the tongue-tie is felt to be causing problems with breastfeeding the child should be referred for a frenotomy.[8]

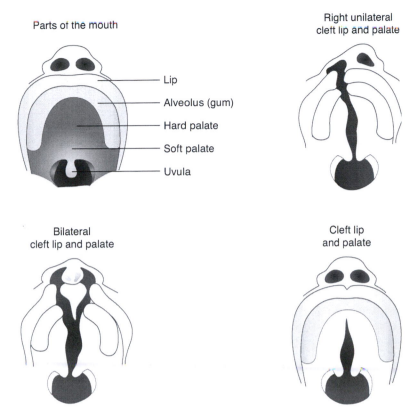

Parts of the mouth

- Lip
- Alveolus (gum)
- Hard palate
- Soft palate
- Uvula

Right unilateral
cleft lip and palate

Bilateral
cleft lip and palate

Cleft lip
and palate

Figure 3 Diagram of cleft lip and palate. Based on images courtesy of Cleft Lip & Palate Association (CLAPA).[10]

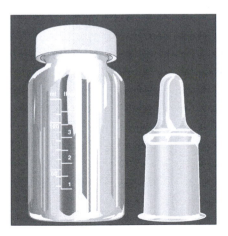

Figure 4 Haberman feeder. Based on images courtesy of Cleft Lip & Palate Association (CLAPA).[10]

Cleft lip and palate

Background

A cleft lip or palate is found in 1 in 500–550 births.[9] It can either be an isolated defect or can be associated with any one of a large number of underlying syndromes such as Pierre Robin or DiGeorge syndrome. This is often a distressing diagnosis for the parents because of its appearance. It can cause the infant a number of problems in the newborn period particularly with feeding.

History and examination

➤ Enquire about any abnormalities on the anomaly scan and if there is any family history of cleft lip or palate.

➤ Enquire about any medication taken by the mother during the pregnancy, e.g. anticonvulsants.

➤ A full systemic examination should be performed by an experienced paediatrician looking for other dysmorphic features or congenital malformations.

Management

➤ This can be a very distressing diagnosis for the parents particularly when the condition has not been diagnosed antenatally. It is useful to show them examples of pre- and post-operation photographs of other children with the same condition.

➤ Give parents information leaflets and advice about support groups.[10]

➤ The child should be referred to the cleft team which usually involves a plastic surgeon and a paediatric dentist.

➤ Support regarding feeding is often required. This may involve a speech and language therapist assessment and the use of special bottles/teats.

➤ Consider sending chromosomes and organising a genetics referral.

➤ Surgical repair of the lip is usually done first around three months of age with the cleft palate being repaired around 9–12 months of age, but this may vary from centre to centre.[9]

Fractured clavicle

Checking the clavicles for fractures should be part of the first postnatal check in the delivery suite. Signs that the clavicle may be fractured include asymmetrical movement of the arms, an asymmetrical Moro reflex and a step or crepitus felt on palpation over the clavicle. Fractured clavicles are more likely in large babies who have had difficult deliveries, e.g. shoulder dystocia.

History and examination

➤ Inspect the clavicles and arms at rest for any obvious deformity or asymmetry.

➤ Palpate over both clavicles for any irregularity.

➤ Check the Moro reflex, looking for evidence of an associated Erb's palsy.

Management

➤ If there are any concerns that the clavicle could be fractured, order a chest radiograph. Although this will generally not alter your management it may be important medico-legally.

➤ The fracture generally heals very quickly in around 7–10 days without any intervention.[7]

➤ Analgesia can be provided with paracetamol at an appropriate dose on an as-required basis.

➤ Immobilising the arm by pinning the infant's sleeve to the body of the baby-grow can also provide pain relief.[7]

➤ Organise outpatient follow-up.

Erb's palsy

This is the most common form of brachial plexus injury in the newborn affecting the C5 and C6 nerve roots. It is most commonly seen in difficult births in big babies, e.g. shoulder dystocia. Here traction on the head and neck during delivery can stretch the nerve roots of the branchial plexus. It can also be associated with clavicular fractures.

History and examination

➤ Inspect the arms for asymmetrical arm movements. Often the affected arm will be held in the classical 'waiter's tip' position with the arm adducted and pronated.

➤ The Moro, biceps and supinator reflexes will often be asymmetrical, but the grasp reflex should be preserved on the affected side.

➤ Examine the clavicles, shoulder and arm to exclude a fracture.

Management

➤ Consider radiography of the upper arm and shoulder if there are any concerns regarding the possibility of a bony injury.

➤ If the infant has respiratory distress a chest radiograph should be performed to exclude an associated phrenic nerve palsy.

➤ Parents are often very anxious that the effects will be permanent. They should be reassured that generally the infant should make a full recovery within weeks or months.[11]

➤ Refer the baby for outpatient physiotherapy to prevent contractures.

➤ Arrange outpatient follow-up. If recovery is limited neurophysiological studies and nerve reconstruction surgery may be required.

Single palmar crease

Single palmar creases can be associated with genetic syndromes such as trisomy 21 and fetal alcohol syndrome but are most often found in healthy individuals without any underlying syndrome. If an infant is found to have unilateral or bilateral single palmar creases, a careful search for other dysmorphic features should be made. In the absence of other dysmorphic features, this can be regarded as a normal variant and no further investigation is required.

History and examination

➤ Enquire about a family history of single palmar creases and maternal alcohol use during the pregnancy.

➤ Examine the infant for dysmorphic features.

Management

➤ If no dysmorphic features are found, reassure the parents that this is a normal variant and no further investigations are required.

➤ If other dysmorphic features are present seek senior advice as the baby will require a genetics workup.

Breast swelling

Breast swelling can occur in both male and female newborns. It is due to the physiological response of maternal hormones on the breast tissue. Sometimes a milky substance, 'witch's milk', can be seen leaking from the nipples.

History and examination

➤ Differentiate simple breast enlargement from mastitis or abscess formation by looking for evidence of erythema, tenderness and increased temperature over the swelling. In the case of an abscess the swelling may also be fluctuant.

Management

➤ In the case of simple breast swelling, reassurance of the parents with an explanation of why this occurs is all that is required.

➤ In the case of mastitis insert an intravenous line and send blood for full blood picture, C-reactive protein and blood culture. Intravenous antibiotics should be started, providing cover against *Staphylococcus aureus,* e.g. flucloxacillin.

➤ If there is no improvement or deterioration on antibiotics, or if there is evidence of a fluctuant swelling at any stage, a paediatric surgical opinion should be sought as either needle aspiration or incision and drainage may be required.

Heart murmurs

Congenital heart disease affects about 1% of all babies. Cardiovascular system (CVS) examination is performed routinely during the neonatal discharge examination with the aim of detecting undiagnosed congenital heart disease. It is important to remember that as a screening tool the CVS examination is neither very sensitive, nor very specific. The aim is to detect as many important conditions as possible, whilst at the same time acknowledging that you won't pick up every one, that most will be relatively minor and that many cardiac murmurs are innocent. Information must be imparted to the parents in a way that acknowledges these facts, whilst at the same time avoiding anxiety. The screening cardiovascular examination is not focused on making anatomical diagnoses, but rather on deciding which babies need further investigation and how quickly this should take place. The main components are checking colour, palpation and auscultation of precordium and checking femoral pulses.

History and examination

➤ Enquire about antenatal ultrasound results – 'Were all your scans during pregnancy reassuring?'

➤ Enquire about family history of congenital heart disease – 'Did you, your partner, or any of his/her siblings have any problems with their heart as a baby?' Usually the answer is no – if yes, check with the cardiologist whether or not referral is needed for echocardiography.

➤ Auscultation of the precordium should take place early in the baby check, before the infant becomes disturbed and cries.

1 Check for cyanosis – if in doubt measure SpO_2.

2 Palpate precordium for thrills/heaves.

3 Auscultate over fourth interspace, lower left sternal border. If a murmur is present, it will usually be audible here. Count heart rate and confirm normal breathing pattern.

4 Check femoral pulses. (VERY IMPORTANT!)

If a murmur is present – try to determine if it is likely to be innocent, pathological or if there are any worrying signs. This will determine the course of action to be followed next.

1 **Innocent murmurs** – these are hard to hear, usually localised to left sternal border with no associated worrying signs.

2 **Pathological Murmurs** – these are louder, longer, tend to radiate and may or may not be accompanied by worrying signs.

3 **Worrying signs** – these include cyanosis, prolonged capillary refill, heart failure (tachycardia, tachypnoea, hepatomegaly) and absent femoral pulses.

Management

➤ Any baby with worrying signs, with or without a cardiac murmur, should be immediately assessed by a paediatric registrar or consultant and admission to the neonatal intensive care unit (NICU) arranged.

➤ Any baby with what sounds like a pathological murmur without worrying signs should have an ECG and chest radiograph. The registrar/consultant should be asked to review the baby when these are done to determine the need (and speed) of further follow-up.

➤ If a murmur is likely to be innocent then it is reasonable to arrange baby clinic review within a few weeks for repeat auscultation without doing an electrocardiogram (ECG) and chest radiograph. If a registrar is available – ask them to confirm your clinical findings.

Absent femorals

Coarctation of the aorta is relatively common and makes up 5–8% of all congenital heart disease.[12] In view of this the femoral pulses must be examined in every baby as part of their routine baby check.

History and examination

➤ Enquire about any family history of congenital heart disease and ask how well the infant has been feeding.

➤ Ensure the infant is relaxed when you palpate the femoral pulses as you will be very unlikely to feel them if the infant is crying and kicking their legs.

➤ Assess the infant for any of the following – pallor, cyanosis, sweating, tachypnoea, cold peripheries or prolonged capillary refill time (normal <2 seconds).

➤ Perform a full cardiovascular examination noting whether or not there is a murmur, whether the heart sounds are normal, the position of the apex beat and whether there are any heaves or thrills.

➤ Check four limb blood pressures. In coarctation of the aorta the blood pressure distal to the site of the coarctation will be lower than proximal to the coarctation. This results in the blood pressure in the arms being higher than the legs (the opposite of what is normally found). Many people regard a difference of 20 mmHg to be significant although studies have shown that this difference is more likely to be found due to variability in measurement rather than coarctation.[13]

➤ Check pre-ductal and post-ductal saturations. Pre-ductal saturations can be checked on the right arm and post-ductal saturations on either of the legs. If there is shunting of deoxygenated blood from right to left across a patent ductus arteriosus the post-ductal saturations will be lower than the pre-ductal saturations.

Management

➤ If there is any doubt regarding whether the femoral pulses are impalpable or weak a senior opinion must be sought without delay.

➤ If the infant appears unwell at the time of examination or if absent femoral pulses are confirmed by a senior, the infant should be admitted to the neonatal unit at once as a prostaglandin infusion is likely to be required to keep the ductus arteriosus patent.

➤ A chest radiograph will be useful to look at heart size and pulmonary vascularity, while an electrocardiogram (ECG) will show any hypertrophy. Echocardiography will be required to confirm the diagnosis.

Abnormal hips

Developmental dysplasia of the hip (DDH) has an incident of 1–2/1000 babies.[14] Untreated, it can result in significant morbidity in later life with limp and limb pain. It is more common in the first-born infant, has a higher incident in girls than boys and affects the left hip more commonly than the right. All infants should be assessed clinically for the condition on routine neonatal discharge examination. This involves looking for risk factors for DDH on history and carrying out a clinical examination of the neonate.

History and examination

➤ Assess for the presence of risk factors for DDH, e.g. family history of DDH, breech presentation at delivery, torticollis or fixed talipes.

➤ Ensure the legs appear to be of equal length and compare both anterior and posterior skin creases for asymmetry.

➤ Perform Ortolani's test by laying the infant on their back with the hip flexed to 90 degrees. Rest your index and middle finger over the infant's greater trochanter and your thumb on the inner aspect of the upper leg. Gently abduct the hip while applying pressure with your fingers over the greater trochanter. This test aims to pick up a dislocated hip and it is positive if you feel a clunk during the test as the femoral head relocates into the acetabulum. You can remember what this test does as Ortolani starts with an O and ends with an I. During the test you are trying to move a hip that is Out back Into the acetabulum.

➤ Perform Barlow's manoeuvre with your hand in the same position, but this time press posteriorly with the palm of your hand and as you adduct the hip apply lateral pressure with your thumb. Here you are looking for a dislocatable hip and the test is positive if you feel movement of the femoral head sliding out of the acetabulum.

➤ The baby should be relaxed throughout the tests, otherwise the risk of a false negative test is significantly increased.

➤ Warn the parents about what you are about to do and explain that the baby might not like the test and may cry.

➤ Shortly after birth there is often a high degree of laxity in the ligaments of the hips. This can cause a click to be felt when the hips are examined. This is not a sign of DDH and the majority of clicks will disappear by two weeks of age if ligament laxity is the cause.

Management

➤ If there are any risk factors for developmental dysplasia of the hip the infant should be referred for an ultrasound scan of both hips, even if the clinical examination is normal.

➤ 'Clicky hips' with no evidence of instability should be brought back to the review clinic in around two weeks' time for repeat examination.[15] If the hip exam is normal at this stage no further action is needed. If there is any concern with the hip exam at this stage refer the baby for an ultrasound scan of both hips, although individual policies may vary from centre to centre.

➤ If Ortolani's or Barlow's test are positive refer the baby urgently for orthopaedic assessment. Do not delay referral by waiting for an ultrasound scan to confirm clinical findings.

Two-cord vessels

When applying the cord clamp in delivery, all infants should have their umbilical cords examined to ensure that there are three vessels present, i.e. two umbilical arteries and one vein. In about 1% of cases only two vessels will be found and there will be a single umbilical artery.[16] The presence of a single umbilical artery may be associated with a higher incidence of other congenital abnormalities and genetic syndromes, although there is still some debate over this.

History and examination

➤ Examine the infant closely, looking for any dysmorphic features or other congenital abnormalities.

Management

➤ If the infant has other abnormalities or dysmorphic features consult with a senior colleague as the infant will need a workup, looking for associated chromosomal abnormalities and congenital malformations particularly involving the cardiovascular, renal and gastrointestinal system.

➤ For the infant without any other abnormalities or dysmorphic features there is no need to send blood for chromosome analysis or to perform investigations to look for occult congenital abnormalities apart from the renal system.

➤ About 8% of infants with a single umbilical artery will have an underlying renal malformation, with a significant proportion of such infants having grade II vesicoureteral reflux or worse.[17] For this reason organising an ultrasound scan of the kidneys and renal tracts combined with a micturating cystourethrogram would be appropriate.

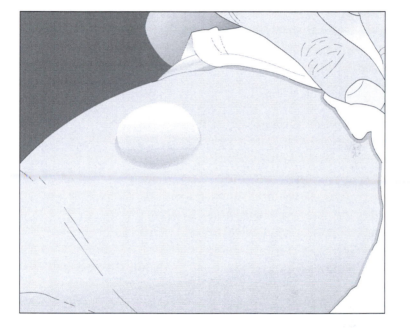

Figure 5 Umbilical hernia. Based on images courtesy of Newborn Services, Auckland City Hospital.[18]

Umbilical hernia

An umbilical hernia is relatively common and occurs due to a gap in the fascia just below the umbilicus. It very rarely becomes obstructed and in the majority of cases will resolve without any intervention before the age of two years. In general it is not related on any other condition but it can be associated with trisomy 21 and congenital hypothyroidism, and it is more common in preterm infants.

History and examination

➤ Ensure that the hernia is easily reducible and that the rest of the abdominal examination is normal. In particular ensure that there are no abdominal masses as increased intra-abdominal pressure can cause an umbilical hernia.

➤ Exclude trisomy 21 and congenital hypothyroidism by clinical examination.

Management

➤ Parents should be advised that the majority of umbilical hernias will resolve by two years of age without intervention.

➤ They should seek medical advice if the hernia appears painful.

➤ If not settling by two years of age, or if the hernia is enlarging or causing the child discomfort, the general practitioner should refer the child for paediatric surgical assessment.

Divarication of the recti

This is a relatively common congenital abnormality where the superior rectus abdominis muscles don't meet in the midline at the linea alba. This is purely a cosmetic abnormality and does not result in any functional problem for the neonate.

History and examination

➤ Perform a full abdominal examination of the neonate.

➤ A bulging can be noted between the rectus muscles over the centre of the abdomen that should be soft. It can be made more prominent by flexing the infant's head.

Management

➤ A simple explanation and reassurance of the parents that it will not result in any functional problem is all that is required.

Inguinal hernia

An inguinal hernia presents as groin swelling in the newborn infant. In the majority of cases the hernia is an indirect hernia occurring due to the presence of a patent processus vaginalis. It is much more common in preterm infants and has a high rate of obstruction if untreated.

History and examination

➤ Examine the groin swelling. You should not be able to get above the swelling and it may increase in size when the infant strains or cries. The hernia may mildly transilluminate if it contains bowel.

➤ Exclude any tenderness on palpation and try to gently reduce the hernia.

Management

➤ Due to the high rate of obstruction an inguinal hernia will need surgical repair.

➤ Discuss with a paediatric surgeon.

➤ If the hernia is tender or irreducible at any stage an urgent paediatric surgical opinion should be sought.

Undescended testes

This is a relatively common problem detected on routine postnatal discharge. The testes develop along the posterior abdominal wall and descend down to the scrotum via the inguinal canal. They are often not fully descended at the time of birth. This occurs more commonly in premature babies, but is found in 2–3% of normal term male infants. As neonates have an active cremasteric reflex the testes can often be retracted into the entrance of the inguinal canal on examination.

History and examination

➤ If the testes are not in the scrotum, palpate both inguinal canals and document findings in child's 'red book' (PHCR).

➤ Ensure the rest of the genitalia is normal and there are no other dysmorphic features.

Management

➤ No need for routine outpatients review.

➤ Ask the general practitioner to re-assess for descent as many will descend over the first year.

➤ The general practitioner should be asked to refer the child to the paediatric surgeons if there is no descent of the testes by around three months of age. This will allow for timely assessment by the paediatric surgeons and if required orchidopexy can be scheduled for around one year of age.

➤ If there is any concern that the infant may have ambiguous genitalia ask for a senior opinion immediately. This is because ambiguous genitalia can be a feature of an endocrine disorder such as congenital adrenal hyperplasia.

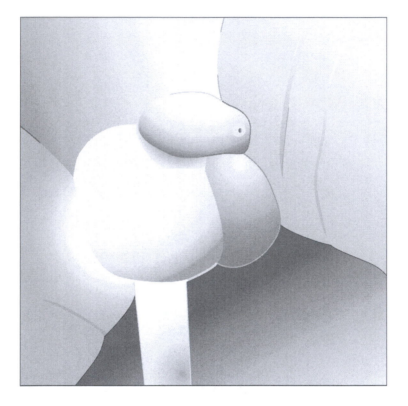

Figure 6 Transillumination of a hydrocele. Based on images courtesy of Newborn Services, Auckland City Hospital.[18]

Hydroceles

A hydrocele is a common finding in the newborn male. It simply represents residual fluid in the processus vaginalis. There are two main forms of hydrocele – a communication hydrocele and a non-communicating hydrocele – but you don't need to be able to clinically differentiate between the two main forms as the initial treatment is the same.

History and examination

➤ Examine the scrotum and inguinal regions for swelling. You must exclude a hydrocele from more serious, but less common, causes of neonatal scrotal swelling such as inguinal hernias, neonatal torsion and testicular neoplasms.

➤ If the swelling is a hydrocele you should be able to get above it, it should transilluminate brightly, it should be non-tender and there should be no discoloration of the surrounding skin.

➤ Document all the above findings and make a comment about the descent of both testes.

Management

➤ The parents should be reassured that this is a common neonatal finding that often resolves without intervention over the first year of life.

➤ They should seek medical advice in the unlikely event of the swelling enlarging or becoming red and tender.

➤ If an uncomplicated hydrocele persists by the age of 2–3 years the child should be referred to a paediatric surgeon.

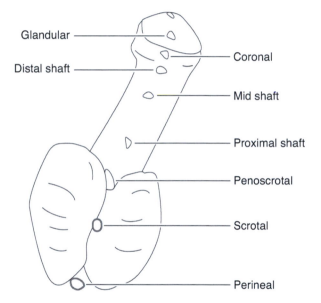

Figure 7 Different positions of urethral meatus in hypospadias.

Hypospadias

This is an abnormality of the male external genitalia in which the urethral meatus opens onto the ventral surface of the penis. When the urethral meatus opens onto the dorsal aspect of the penis it is called epispadias. Hypospadias is the most common penile abnormality, occurring in 3 per 1000 boys. Hypospadias occurs due to arrest in the development of the urethra, foreskin and ventral parts of the penis. There can be an abnormal fibrous band or chordee on the ventral aspect of the penis, which can result in bowing of the penis. The urethral meatus may be found on the ventral aspect of the penis, on the glans, coronal sulcus, shaft of penis, scrotum or perineum.

In about 10% of cases there may be unilateral or bilateral cryptorchidism. When hypospadias is associated with cryptorchidism the infant should be investigated for possible intersex anomaly.

History and examination

➤ Check whether baby has passed urine and also enquire about urinary stream as there may be associated meatal stenosis.

➤ Note the position of the urethral meatus and the presence of a chordee. The prepuce may be incompletely formed.

Management

➤ Make a routine outpatient referral to a paediatric urologist.

➤ If the urethral meatus is positioned in the proximal, penoscrotal, scrotal or perineal position or if there is associated cryptorchidism, organise an ultrasound scan of the renal tracts to look for associated abnormalities.[19]

➤ Severe hypospadias associated with unilateral or bilateral impalpable testes or ambiguous genitalia will require an urgent genetic and endocrine workup to exclude intersex, e.g. congenital adrenal hyperplasia.

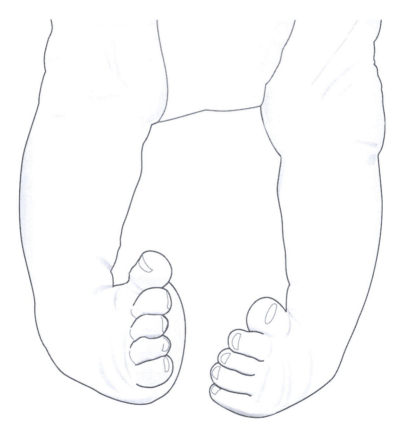

Figure 8 Talipes equinovarus. Courtesy of Daniel J Hatch, DPM,FACFAS.[20]

Talipes

Positional talipes equinus deformity is relatively common and is due to the position of the baby in the uterus. In the majority of cases this will return to normal with no action. The baby may require stretching to help this process, with input from a physiotherapist.

History and examination

Assess whether the talipes is positional or not. If you are able to invert and evert the foot passively by applying gentle pressure, it is positional. If not, it is fixed.

Management

➤ Refer for physiotherapy assessment if positional.

➤ Fixed talipes equinovarus or talipes calcaneovalgus deformity should be referred to orthopaedics as a matter of urgency.

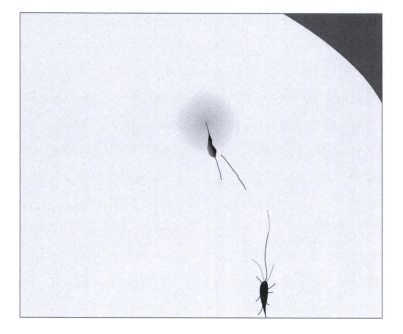

Figure 9 A sacral dimple. Based on images courtesy of Newborn Services, Auckland City Hospital.[22]

Sacral dimple

Spinal dimples are a common finding. In the majority of cases they are simple dimples (<5 mm deep in the midline and <25 mm from the anus).[21] These simple dimples are not associated with any underlying spinal abnormality; no further investigation is necessary and the parents can be reassured that this is a normal variant found in up to 4% of the population.[21] However, if the sacral dimple is large (>5 mm deep) or located more than 25 mm from the anal verge it may be associated with occult spinal dysraphism.[21] The risk of occult spinal dysraphism is also increased by the presence of lumbosacral lipomas, hairy patches, skin tags or vascular lesions.[21] The presence of more than one cutaneous lesion overlying the spine significantly increases the risk of occult spinal dysraphism.[21]

History and examination

➤ Document the size and position of the dimple in relation to the midline and the anal margin.

➤ Look for any associated spinal abnormalities such as a lumbosacral lipoma, hairy patch, skin tag or vascular lesion.

➤ Examine the rest of the spine to ensure it looks normal.

➤ Examine the position, tone, power and reflexes in the lower limbs.

➤ Enquire about whether the infant has had any difficulty passing urine or opening their bowels.

Management

➤ If the dimple is <5 mm in the midline and <25 mm from the anal margin and no other spinal abnormality is present, reassure the parents that this is a normal variant and no further investigation is necessary.

➤ If the dimple is atypical (e.g. >5 mm and >25 mm from the anal margin) the patient should be referred for a spinal ultrasound scan.

➤ If there is a lumbosacral lipoma, hairy patch, skin tag or vascular lesion, the infant should also be referred for ultrasound imaging of the spine.

Bruising

The birth process can often be traumatic for the baby and it is not uncommon to find evidence of bruising. This is particularly true when the infant has been born instrumentally, e.g. forceps or ventouse. All bruising noted at delivery should be documented and when bruising can't be explained or is excessive, other causes should be looked for.

History and examination

➤ Enquire about the mode of birth. Was it difficult? Were forceps or a ventouse required?

➤ Were all the bruises present at birth or are new bruises forming?

➤ Has the infant had vitamin K?

➤ Check the mother's notes for a recent platelet count, her blood group and for the presence of antibodies.

➤ Enquire about a family history of haematological disorders, e.g. haemophilia, von Willebrand disease or maternal idiopathic thrombocytopenia.

➤ Perform a full systemic examination of the neonate, documenting the presence and size of all bruises. Pay particular attention to the abdominal system, looking for evidence of hepatosplenomegaly.

Management

➤ Minor bruising or bruising that can be explained (e.g. in the shape of a ventouse cup or forceps blade) needs explanation to the parents and reassurance that it should settle quickly.

➤ If the bruising is large the infant will be at a slightly higher risk of jaundice and there should be a low threshold for checking the serum bilirubin if the infant appears jaundiced.

➤ If there is multiple or large bruising that can't be explained, have a low threshold for checking a full blood picture and coagulation screen and discussing any abnormalities with your senior.

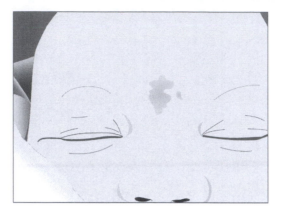

Figure 10 Salmon patches. Based on images courtesy of Newborn Services, Auckland City Hospital.[23]

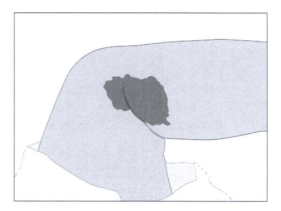

Figure 11 Strawberry naevus. Based on images courtesy of Newborn Services, Auckland City Hospital.[23]

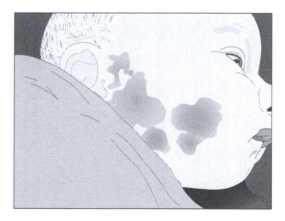

Figure 12 Port wine stain. Based on images courtesy of Newborn Services, Auckland City Hospital.[23]

Birthmarks

There are a number of common birthmarks you will be asked to review. Probably the most common are salmon patches. These are pink macular marks most commonly found over the back of the neck (stork mark) and over the eyelids (angel kisses). In general the marks over the eyelids fade with time and the ones on the back of the neck either fade or become covered with hair.

A strawberry naevus or cavernous haemangioma is not usually present at birth but develops over the first few weeks. Its natural history is that it tends to get bigger over the first year of life before slowly regressing. It doesn't need any treatment unless it is obstructing the eye, as there is a risk of amblyopia. If it is overlying the spine an underlying occult spinal dysraphism should be excluded by ultrasound.

Port wine stains are permanent birthmarks that are much redder in colour than stork marks. When a port wine stain occurs on the face, most commonly over the upper division of the trigeminal nerve, Sturge–Weber syndrome should be excluded.

History and examination

Document the shape, size and position of the birthmark.

Management

➤ The natural course of the naevus should be explained to the parents.

➤ A port wine stain should be referred to dermatology as laser treatment may be required.

➤ If you are unsure about what a particular birthmark is, ask for a senior opinion.

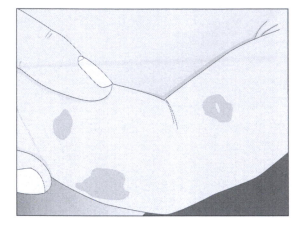

Figure 13 Rash of erythema toxicum.

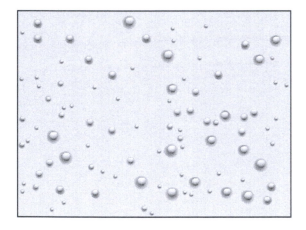

Figure 14 Transient pustular melanosis. Based on images courtesy of Newborn Services, Auckland City Hospital.[27]

Rashes

Erythema toxicum neonatorum and transient pustular melanosis are the two most common neonatal rashes you will be asked to review. Although they are both harmless there may be parental anxiety surrounding the rash, so you must be able to make a confident diagnosis and offer reassurance.

History and examination

➤ With any neonatal rash ask about when it was first noted – was it present at birth or did it develop later? Erythema toxicum tends to present within the first four days, but is rarely present at birth.[24] Transient neonatal pustular melanosis is always present at birth.[25]

➤ Ask about a maternal history of infections during the pregnancy, e.g. herpes simplex and varicella.

➤ Describe the rash. Erythema toxicum is a generalised rash with a background of erythematous macules combined with papules, vesicles and pustules.[24]

The rash of transient neonatal pustular melanosis appears in three stages. First, there are small non-erythematous pustules which rupture easily. Next an area of white scale develop around the pustule and finally a central brown macule develops.[26]

➤ Ensure the infant is clinically well by performing a full systemic examination, in particular looking for evidence of sepsis.

Management

➤ The parents should be reassured that both these common rashes are self-limiting and no treatment is required. The rash of erythema toxicum and the vesicles and pustules in neonatal pustular melanosis should disappear by around 4–7 days of age, while the macules in neonatal pustular melanosis can take a few months to disappear.

➤ If you are unable to make a confident clinical diagnosis or don't feel the rash you are seeing fits with either of these rashes, ask for a senior review.

3. Clinical Problems

Respiratory distress

A newborn baby should have a respiratory rate between 40 and 60 breaths per minute. Signs of respiratory distress include tachypnoea, indrawing, recession, nasal flaring and moaning/grunting. The moaning or grunting is heard at the end of expiration and represents the infant trying to increase its positive end expiratory pressure (PEEP).

There are often clues in the history that will help you decide on the likely cause of respiratory distress. Transient tachypnoea of the newborn (TTN) is probably the most common. It represents lung fluid that hasn't been resorbed yet and is more common in babies born by caesarean section. Preterm babies can have respiratory distress syndrome (RDS) due to surfactant deficiency. Pneumothorax is more common after positive pressure ventilation in delivery suite, and if there has been meconium staining the baby can have meconium aspiration syndrome. Occasionally babies can have problems such as diaphragmatic hernias; however, with routine antenatal scanning, undiagnosed diaphragmatic hernias are thankfully a rare occurrence.

Other problems outside the respiratory systems can cause respiratory distress in the newborn. These include sepsis (respiratory compensation for a metabolic acidosis), polycythaemia and cardiac problems causing heart failure.

History and examination

➤ Enquire about the method of delivery. TTN is more common after caesarean section.

➤ Were there any risk factors for sepsis? This increases the risk of congenital pneumonia.

➤ Was there meconium stained liquor or fetal distress? This increases the risk of meconium aspiration syndrome.

➤ Did the baby need any resuscitation? Resuscitation using positive pressure ventilation can increase the risk of pneumothorax.

➤ What is the gestation of the baby? RDS is more common in preterm infants and infants of diabetic mothers. If the baby was under 34 weeks were antenatal steroids given?

➤ Were there any abnormalities seen on the antenatal scans (e.g. diaphragmatic hernia, oligohydramnios, which can cause pulmonary hypoplasia), or cardiac abnormalities?

➤ Check the infant's observations, i.e. pulse, respiratory rate, oxygen saturations, temperature, capillary refill time and level of consciousness.

➤ Perform a full systemic examination particularly focusing on the respiratory system. Look for signs of respiratory distress, check that chest wall movement and air entry are symmetrical (may be asymmetrical in a pneumothorax or congenital pneumonia). Are there any added sounds?

➤ Ensure you have examined the cardiovascular system including palpating the femoral pulses and looking for evidence of heart failure (associated tachycardia, hepatomegaly, cold peripheries and sweating).

Management

➤ For the well infant with mild respiratory distress, normal oxygen saturations and no unilateral signs, it is appropriate to monitor the infant in an incubator in the delivery suite with regular observations and repeated paediatric review after an hour. If the infant has TTN it will often make some improvement over the first few hours but should not deteriorate. As this is the most common cause of respiratory distress in the newborn, by managing the infant in this way you can avoid unnecessary neonatal unit admissions. However, if on repeat review there are signs of deterioration, e.g. increasing respiratory distress, development of an oxygen requirement, then ask for a senior review as a chest radiograph and admission to the neonatal unit may be required.

➤ Remember that a healthy newborn infant will have oxygen saturations of around 70% at birth. It takes on average about 15 minutes to reach levels of 95% in a normal healthy infant, but can take up to an hour.[28] With this in mind your management of a well newborn infant with mild respiratory distress, no worrying signs, but low oxygen saturation will depend on the timing after birth. In the first hour of birth, borderline saturation can be attributed to normal neonatal physiology, so it is reasonable to observe the neonate in delivery suite and administer incubator oxygen as required. If there is any deterioration (increasing respiratory distress or increasing oxygen requirements) or an ongoing oxygen requirement after the first hour, a senior opinion should be sought and neonatal unit admission considered.

➤ If the infant is unwell, has more than mild respiratory distress or there are signs of a pneumothorax, meconium aspiration syndrome or congenital pneumonia, ask for a senior opinion at once.

Cyanosis

You will often be asked to see babies who appear cyanosed shortly after birth. The important thing here is to differentiate peripheral cyanosis, which is relatively common, from central cyanosis, which can be potentially serious. In peripheral cyanosis the infant is peripherally blue but its lips and tongue are pink. This is due to poor perfusion of the peripheries and is relatively common in the immediate postnatal period. In central cyanosis both the peripheries and the lips and tongue are blue. This represents an increased amount of deoxygenated haemoglobin in the blood. If you are unsure whether the cyanosis is peripheral or central check the SpO2.

When interpreting the oxygen saturation in the newborn it is important to have a basic understanding of normal neonatal physiology. At birth a healthy newborn infant will have oxygen saturations of around 70%. It takes on average about 15 minutes to reach a level of 95%, although this process can take up to an hour in a normal healthy infant.[28]

Also at birth the pressures in the pulmonary circulation are higher than in an older infant. The presence of a patent ductus arteriosus (PDA) means that deoxygenated blood can shunt from right to left across the PDA. For this reason, to get an accurate recording of the oxygen saturations in the newborn it is best to check pre-ductal saturation by placing the saturation probe on the right hand.

In the majority of cases, low oxygen saturations or central cyanosis will mean a respiratory problem, particularly if combined with signs of respiratory distress. Low oxygen saturations or central cyanosis with minimal signs of respiratory distress, or which is unresponsive to oxygen therapy should be regarded as congenital cyanotic heart disease until proven otherwise.

History and examination

➤ Enquire about risk factors for respiratory conditions, e.g. preterm (respiratory distress syndrome), delivered by caesarean section (TTN), meconium stained liquor (MAS), resuscitation required in delivery suite (pneumothorax) and risk factors for sepsis (congenital pneumonia).

➤ Enquire about risk factors for congenital heart disease, e.g. abnormal heart on the antenatal ultrasound scan and family history of congenital heart disease.

➤ Examine the infant's lips and tongue to determine if the cyanosis is peripheral or central.

➤ If the cyanosis is peripheral check the infant's temperature and central perfusion by checking capillary refill time over the sternum (normal <2 seconds).

➤ For central cyanosis perform a full systemic examination focusing on the cardiovascular and respiratory systems (heart murmurs, heaving or displaced apex beat, femoral pulses, signs of respiratory distress and focal respiratory signs).

Management

➤ In peripheral cyanosis with normal oxygen saturations and good central perfusion (central CRT <2 seconds) offer an explanation to the parents and advice about keeping the infant warm. If the infant is poorly perfused centrally ask for a senior opinion at once and manage the infant as per the septic infant.

➤ For infants with central cyanosis or true low oxygen saturations administer oxygen and ask for an urgent senior opinion as neonatal unit admission for further investigation/management will likely be required.

Tachycardia

The normal range for the term neonate's heart rate is 120–160 beats per minute. When the infant is unsettled the heart rate may go above 160 temporarily, but a persistent heart rate greater than 160 beats per minute requires further evaluation. Causes of an elevated heart rate include pain, pyrexia, sepsis, dehydration, thyrotoxicosis, substance withdrawal and cardiac arrhythmias such as supraventricular tachycardia (SVT). SVT must be excluded if the heart rate is greater than 220.

History and examination

➤ Enquire about the antenatal anomaly scan and whether the heart rate was normal during the pregnancy.

➤ Were there any risk factors for sepsis, any maternal medicines or drug use during the pregnancy or a maternal history of a thyroid disorder?

➤ Perform a full set of observations including heart rate, oxygen saturations, respiratory rate, temperature and capillary refill time.

➤ Perform a full systemic examination, in particular looking at the cardiovascular system, checking for any signs of trauma from delivery that may be causing the infant pain, signs of sepsis or meningitis and signs of dehydration.

Management

➤ Management of the tachycardia should be directed towards the likely underlying cause identified from examination.

➤ For persistent tachycardia greater than 160 consider sepsis. Have a low threshold for performing a limited septic screen (full blood picture, C-reactive protein and blood culture) and starting the baby on antibiotics.

➤ A 12-lead ECG should be performed to exclude a tachydysrhythmia.

➤ If the tachycardia is combined with signs of poor perfusion (e.g. CRT >2 seconds) administer a 10 ml/kg bolus of 0.9% sodium chloride and arrange for neonatal unit admission.

➤ If the heart rate is greater than 220 it should be regarded as SVT until proven otherwise. This is a medical emergency and you should request the urgent presence of your senior while you manage the baby using the ABC approach.

Bradycardia

The normal range for the term neonate's heart rate is 120–160 beats per minute. It is, however, normal for the resting heart rate to dip below this when the baby is very settled or sleeping. However, you would then expect an increase in the heart rate when you disturb the infant to examine him/her. Causes of a persistently low heart rate include hypothermia, hypoxic-ischaemic encephalopathy, hypothyroidism and cardiac arrhythmias such as heart block, which can be associated with maternal systemic lupus erythematosus (SLE).

History and examination

➤ Enquire about the antenatal anomaly scan and whether the heart rate was normal during the pregnancy.

➤ Is there a maternal history of thyroid disorders or SLE?

➤ Were there any risk factors for HIE (e.g. low cord pH, prolonged period of resuscitation)?

➤ Perform a full set of observations including heart rate, saturations, respiratory rate, temperature and capillary refill time.

➤ Perform a full systemic examination, in particular looking at the cardiovascular system as to whether the heart rate appears regular or whether there are any missed beats.

Management

➤ Recording a 12-lead ECG is mandatory and this should be reviewed with your senior or a paediatric cardiologist.

➤ Further management will depend on the cause of the bradycardia.

➤ If there is any evidence that the infant is not tolerating the bradycardia (e.g. prolonged capillary refill time) this is a medical emergency and you should initially manage the baby using the ABC approach.

Sepsis

As the mortality rate for untreated neonatal sepsis can be as high as 50%,[29] assessing and managing babies with risk factors for, or possible signs of sepsis, is probably the most important job you will undertake on the postnatal wards.

The two biggest risk factors for sepsis in the neonate are maternal carriage of group B streptococcus (GBS) and prolonged rupture of membranes (PROM). About 30% of women are colonised with GBS at the time of delivery, but only 2 in 1000 neonates develop GBS sepsis.[29] If the mother had a previous infant affected by GBS sepsis, this significantly increases the risk of infection to the neonate.

The definition of prolonged rupture of membranes varies widely, but in general if membranes have been ruptured for more than 24 hours you can regard the neonate as having an increased risk of infection. This risk is at its highest if the mother has associated chorioamnionitis, e.g. maternal pyrexia, increased inflammatory markers, uterine tenderness or foul smelling discharge/amniotic fluid.

Other risk factors that predispose the neonate to sepsis include being preterm (reduced immune response) and maternal urinary tract infection/ positive vaginal swabs at the time of delivery. If there is evidence of maternal GBS or chorioamnionitis many hospitals will give the mother prophylactic antibiotic in labour to reduce the risk of transmission of infection to the baby. To be effective these antibiotics need to be given at least 4 hours prior to delivery and if this is not the case you should regard the baby's risk of sepsis as being higher than if the antibiotic coverage was adequate.

Another important area to cover here is how to interpret blood results in an infant who has had a septic screen performed. The newborn infant has a higher white cell count that an adult or older child (normal reference range 9–30 10^9/L at birth). In sepsis the white cell count can either be increased or low ($< 9 \times 10^9$/L). Further evidence of sepsis can be gained by looking at the platelet count which is often low in sepsis ($< 150 \times 10^9$/L).

The full blood picture is often taken in conjunction with a C-reactive protein (CRP) measurement. If the CRP is raised at all this provides supporting evidence of established infection in the neonate. However, if the CRP is normal this doesn't exclude infection as many infants with sepsis, will have a normal CRP initially and monitoring trends in the CRP is much more useful than an isolated measurement.

Isolating an organism in the blood culture is the gold standard for confirming neonatal sepsis, although not all babies with sepsis will have positive blood cultures and the blood cultures may take up to 48 hours before you will have a result. However, a negative blood culture in a well baby at 48 hours provides you with some additional evidence to help you decide whether you can stop antibiotics or not, and if positive will help you decide on the duration and type of antibiotics to give.

History and examination

➤ Ask about risk factors for sepsis (e.g. maternal GBS carriage, a sibling with GBS sepsis, prolonged rupture of membranes), whether appropriate antibiotics were given in labour where indicated (>4 hours prior to delivery), maternal pyrexia in labour >38°C, raised inflammatory markers in the mother, maternal uterine tenderness, foul smelling liquor or discharge, positive vaginal swabs and maternal urinary tract infection at the time of delivery.

➤ Look at the baby's observation for evidence of sepsis, e.g. pyrexia, tachycardia, tachypnoea and prolonged capillary refill time. Normal observations in the term infant are recorded below.

Table 1 Normal neonatal observations – reference ranges

Observation	Reference range
Pulse	120–160
Respiratory rate	40–60
Temperature	36.4–37.7°C
Capillary refill time	<2 seconds

➤ Note the mother's temperature at the time of delivery. The well baby's temperature at birth is normally 0.5°C above the mother's temperature.

➤ Perform a full systemic examination of the infant, looking in particular for lethargy, irritability, whether the baby dislikes handling, a tense or bulging anterior fontanelle or erythema round the umbilical cord.

➤ Consider checking the capillary blood glucose in infants suspected of having sepsis as it may be raised due to the release of stress hormones.

Management

In general, a careful history, examination and observation, with a clear plan for the ward staff, are more useful than screening blood tests.[30]

The management of well babies with normal examination and observations, who have risk factors for sepsis, will depend on the gestational age of the baby and the number and type of each risk factor present. You should follow your local hospital guidelines or national guidelines, e.g. NICE guideline on Intrapartum Care covers management of PROM, but a few general principles apply:

1 **High Risk Babies** *(preterm with any risk factors for sepsis, evidence of maternal chorioamnionitis, maternal GBS colonisation combined with inadequate antenatal antibiotics or PROM, a previous sibling with GBS sepsis or baby with multiple risk factors for sepsis).*

— Site an intravenous line, send blood for FBP, CRP and blood culture.

— The baby should be commenced on suitable antibiotics (e.g. intravenous benzylpenicillin and gentamicin) while the results of the blood culture are awaited.

— The well baby will require at least daily paediatric review on the postnatal ward and regular observation, including temperature, pulse, respiratory rate and capillary refill time, should be performed. At a minimum these observations should be recorded shortly after birth, at 1 hour of age, 2 hours of age, and then two hourly for the next 10 hours. If the baby remains well after this the frequency of observations can be reduced.

— Whether the baby gets a prophylactic course of antibiotics (48 hours pending blood culture results) or a treatment course (five days minimum, possibly longer depending on the organism) will depend on the information you have gathered at that stage (initial blood results, blood cultures at 48 hours, clinical condition of the baby while on antibiotics).

2 **Low risk babies** *(term infants with PROM only, term infants with maternal carriage of GBS but adequate antenatal antibiotics or well term babies with one isolated risk factor for sepsis).*

— These babies should have regular observations for the first 12–24 hours. If at any stage there is any concern with the observations or clinical condition of the baby they should be managed as high-risk babies above.

— Some hospital policies may recommend initially performing screening bloods in these babies without starting antibiotics as a slightly less invasive strategy. However, observation is more sensitive than screening blood tests in picking up sepsis. As the blood tests cause pain and distress for both the baby and parents, NICE no longer recommend the routine use of screening bloods in well term babies with isolated PROM.[31]

— Many paediatricians would argue that if you are concerned enough to perform screening bloods on the baby you should cover the baby with 48 hours of antibiotics while the blood cultures are pending.

3 **Babies with abnormal observations or signs of sepsis**

— Regardless of risk factors these babies should have screening bloods performed and be covered with antibiotics.

— You should ask for a senior review as they may want to perform a full septic screen (lumbar puncture and supra-pubic aspiration of urine as well as blood cultures) prior to starting antibiotics.

— Babies with signs of sepsis should be admitted to the neonatal unit for closer monitoring/further management.

Jaundice

Jaundice can be a normal physiological event for the newborn infant, affecting 50–60% of babies over the first week of life. Physiological jaundice accounts for the majority of this and it occurs for a number of reasons. First, at birth the neonate has a high red blood cell count which is no longer required and the newborn's red cells have a much shorter life span than that of an older child. These factors result in a high breakdown of red blood cells over the first few days of life, which in turn produces a large amount of bilirubin. This high bilirubin load combined with immature liver function results in physiological jaundice. It therefore follows that any baby who has a large amount of bruising from delivery or has developed a cephalhaematoma will be at a higher risk of developing jaundice.

Babies who are breastfed can also develop breast milk jaundice. This tends to develop slightly later than physiological jaundice, around day 4–7 and is due to a substance in the breast milk inhibiting the enzyme that conjugates the bilirubin.

Jaundice in the first day of life is always pathological and cannot be attributed to either physiological jaundice or breast milk jaundice.

Causes of jaundice in the first 24 hours include:

1 **Rhesus disease** – This occurs in mothers who are rhesus negative who have a baby who is rhesus positive. The mother has previously acquired antibodies against the baby's rhesus antigen which can cross the placenta and cause the breakdown of the baby's blood cells resulting in anaemia and jaundice. This is now thankfully rare due to the routine use of anti-D. Most hospitals routinely check the blood group and Coombs status on cord blood of babies of rhesus negative mothers. In rhesus disease the Coombs test is strongly positive, indicating a large amount of antibodies attacking the baby's red blood cells. However, the interpretation of a positive Coombs test is complicated by the fact that the routine use of antenatal anti-D often results in a weakly positive Coombs test secondary to the effects of the anti-D rather that rhesus disease itself. This reduces the usefulness of a positive Coombs test in this setting.

2 **ABO incompatibility** – Normally anti-A and anti-B antibodies are IgM and are therefore too large to cross the placenta. Occasionally a mother can have an IgG form of the antibody, which can cross the placenta. This is more commonly anti-A, but occasionally anti-B. This antibody can then attack the baby's red blood cells if they have the corresponding antigen (e.g. anti-A antibody will be able to attack a baby's red blood cells if the blood group is A or AB, but not if it is B or O). This usually results in haemolysis to a less severe degree than rhesus disease and the Coombs test is often weakly positive.

3 **Other antibody reactions** – There are numerous other antibodies that can be present in the mother's blood and that can cross the placenta, causing haemolysis and subsequent jaundice. Again the Coombs test will be positive.

4 **Red blood cell membrane defects** – Hereditary spherocytosis and elliptocytosis result in abnormally shaped cells that have increased fragility and are easily broken down in the spleen. These conditions are inherited. As a mechanical process is responsible for the breakdown of the red blood cell, rather than an antibody reaction, the Coombs test is negative.

5 **Congenital infection** – Congenital infections tend to result in a conjugated hyperbilirubinaemia combined with other signs of congenital infection.

The above list mentions some of the main causes of jaundice in the newborn but is by no means exhaustive and a larger textbook of paediatrics should be referred to for more details on this important topic.

The main reason we worry about hyperbilirubinaemia in the newborn is that high levels of unconjugated (indirect) bilirubin can cross the blood brain barrier and be deposited in the basal ganglia causing acute bilirubin encephalopathy. This can later lead to the development of cerebral palsy and neurosensory deafness. To prevent this it is important to monitor the serum bilirubin in the newborn and intervene prior to the bilirubin reaching a dangerous level. The main method of treating hyperbilirubinaemia is phototherapy. Phototherapy uses light in the blue-green spectrum with wavelength 420–470 nm, which causes a conformational change in the molecular structure of bilirubin, making it water soluble. As a result the bilirubin molecule can no longer pass through the blood brain barrier and is able to be excreted from the body. If the bilirubin level continues to rise under single phototherapy more lights can be added or very infrequently an exchange transfusion may be required to prevent acute bilirubin encephalopathy from developing.

Risk factors for jaundice can be remembered using the mnemonic below:

Jaundice visible in first 24 hours of life.

A sibling with neonatal jaundice or anaemia. Acidosis, Asphyxia.

Unrecognised haemolysis – ABO, Rh, other blood group incompatibility, UDPGtf deficiency (Crigler-Najjar, Gilbert's syndrome).

Non optimal feeding (formula or breastfed).

Deficiency of glucose-6-phosphate dehydrogenase (G6PD).

Infection, Infant of diabetic mother, Immaturity (prematurity).

Cephalhaematoma or bruising, Central haematocrit >65% (polycythaemia).

East Asian, Mediterranean, Native American heritage.

History and examination

➤ Review the mother's notes for blood group and antibody status.

➤ If cord blood has been sent for group and Coombs, review these and compare the baby's blood group to the mother's blood group.

➤ Are there risk factors for sepsis?

➤ Enquire about a family history of a haematological condition (e.g. hereditary spherocytosis, elliptocytosis or G6PD deficiency), all of which can cause jaundice in the first 24 hours.

➤ Enquire about how the infant is feeding. Breastfeeding is associated with jaundice as is dehydration from poor feeding.

➤ Note the gestational age – preterm babies are at higher risk of hyperbilirubinaemia and will require intervention at an earlier stage.

➤ Perform a full systemic examination of the infant. In particular assess the colour for the degree of jaundice or for any evidence of pallor that may indicate haemolysis.

➤ Look for any signs of dehydration (dry mucous membranes or sunken anterior fontanelle), evidence of bruising, signs of sepsis (prolonged capillary refill time, tachycardia, lethargy) or any hepatosplenomegaly on abdominal examination.

Management

➤ If the infant appears more than mildly jaundiced the bilirubin level should be checked using either a transcutaneous bilirubinometer or by measuring a serum bilirubin level.

➤ Use the American Academy of Pediatrics or your departmental nomogram to decide if the infant requires phototherapy.[32]

➤ The result obtained using a transcutaneous bilirubinometer are accurate to within 50 mol/L. If adding 50 mol/L to the result obtained means the infant would require phototherapy and a serum bilirubin should be sent.

➤ For babies who are close to the phototherapy line on the nomogram, but not currently needing phototherapy, it is advisable not to discharge these babies until the trend in repeat bilirubin levels shows that the baby will be unlikely to require phototherapy.

➤ The frequency of repeating the serum bilirubin will depend on the baby's risk factors for jaundice, the rate of rise in the serum bilirubin levels and how high the actual serum bilirubin level is. For a baby who is Coombs positive or has a rapidly rising serum bilirubin level it would be advisable to have a much lower threshold for starting phototherapy and the serum bilirubin may need to be checked four hourly. On the other hand, for a baby who has no risk factors for jaundice, a slow rise in the serum bilirubin levels and who is just in the phototherapy zone, it would be reasonable to leave the baby under phototherapy and check the serum bilirubin in 24 hour's time.

➤ Once phototherapy treatment has begun the rate of rise in total serum bilirubin should be <5 mol/L/hr. A rate of rise of >10 mol/L/hr is of concern and a rise of >14 mol/L/hr is pathological and exchange transfusion should be strongly considered.

➤ Once phototherapy is started it is advisable to leave the baby under phototherapy for a minimum of 24 hours to avoid the need for babies to have a repeated course of phototherapy. A repeat bilirubin level should be checked prior to discontinuing phototherapy to ensure the level has fallen outside the treatment zone. Many doctors would repeat the bilirubin level 8–12 hours after discontinuing phototherapy to ensure that there has not been a rebound in the bilirubin level.

➤ Jaundice is closely related to hydration and an assessment of the infant's feeding must be made. In dehydrated infants, rehydration will usually lead to a prompt decline in serum bilirubin levels. Also phototherapy increases the infant's insensible losses so the baby will actually need slightly more fluid while under phototherapy (around 10% per set of lights).

➤ All infants with more than mild jaundice and every infant with jaundice in the first 24 hours should have a blood group checked and a Coombs test performed. Prior to taking the blood tests check the notes as these tests may have already been performed on cord blood if the mother is rhesus negative.

➤ Any baby who is Coombs positive or is jaundiced within the first 24 hours also needs to have a full blood picture checked, looking at the haemoglobin as the baby is at risk of haemolysis. The baby will also need serial bilirubin checks from an early age and there should be a low threshold for starting phototherapy. If the baby develops a rapidly rising bilirubin don't forget to repeat the full blood picture, as the increase in bilirubin may be combined with a fall in haemoglobin.

➤ If there are any concerns regarding sepsis, have a low threshold for performing screening bloods (full blood picture, C-reactive protein and blood culture) and starting intravenous antibiotics, as jaundice is often present in babies who are septic.

Hypoglycaemia

Low blood sugar is a common and controversial problem in the newborn. Despite the extensive research on neonatal glucose metabolism, no uniformly accepted standards are used to define hypoglycaemia or hyperglycaemia.[33-35] In the fetus a linear relationship is seen between the blood glucose concentration in the mother and that in the fetus. At birth the blood glucose in the newborn is 80–90% of that of the mothers and this trend is seen even if the mother is euglycaemic, hypoglycaemic or hyperglycaemic. In term neonates (>37 weeks' gestation) who weigh between 2500 grams and 4000 grams, the plasma glucose concentration is lowest between 1 and 2 hours of age with a significant rise during the third hour of life.[36] A plasma glucose concentration below 1.9 mmol/L in the first 3 hours of life should be of concern.[36,37] A number of studies have suggested that a blood glucose level below 2.6 mmol/L may be associated with short- and long-term neurological sequelae.[37] For practical purposes hypoglycaemia in neonates is defined as a plasma glucose value below 2.6 mmol/L. Hypoglycaemia can be symptomatic or asymptomatic. Symptomatic hypoglycaemia can be convulsive or non-convulsive. Fifty per cent of neonates with symptomatic convulsive hypoglycaemia and 12% of the symptomatic non-convulsive group can have neurological abnormalities on follow-up compared to 6% of neonates with asymptomatic hypoglycaemia.

Bedside capillary glucose measurement is performed with a glucometer or a HemoCue glucose systems apparatus. These are useful only as a screening device for neonatal hypoglycaemia. A persistently low glucose should always be confirmed with a lab measurement and a cause should always be sought. There are differences between capillary and venous whole blood and plasma glucose values. Whole blood glucose values are lower than plasma glucose values.

Glucose metabolism

In contrast to the adult who is fully independent in respect of nutritional requirements, the fetus is completely dependent on the placental transfer of glucose and other nutrients. The newborn is in a transitional phase between the two states of complete dependence and independence.

For normal cerebral development and function an adequate amount of substrate must be supplied to the brain. In physiological conditions glucose is the primary energy substrate for the human brain. When there is an imbalance in the supply and demand for energy production other organic substances are capable of supplementing glucose.

At birth there is cessation of placental supply of glucose and nutrients and immediately post-birth hepatic stores of glycogen are broken down to maintain reasonable amounts of nutritional support. Glycogen-6-phosphatase is the rate limiting enzyme for hepatic glycogenolysis and it is expressed in low levels in the newborn, increasing to adult levels within a few days after birth. In the interim the body responds with an endocrine stress response involving insulin and glucagon drive hepatic glycogenolysis, lipolysis and free fatty acid oxidation producing lactic acid and ketone bodies as alternate fuel for maintaining cerebral energy metabolism. In preparation for birth there is a doubling of the glycogen stores in the fetus that occurs at 36 weeks' gestation. At birth the plasma insulin level falls and glucagon levels rise markedly, leading to mobilisation of the glycogen stores, which are rapidly depleted within the first 12–24 hours of life. Further maintenance of glucose concentration depends on feeding.

Preterm infants have very poor glycogen stores, the rate limiting enzyme glucose-6-phosphatase is significantly lower than in term infants, and their capability to mount a response with alternative substrates is also impaired, hence being at increased risk to hypoglycaemia in the newborn period. Similarly growth-restricted babies also have functional hyperinsulinism, which predisposes them to hypoglycaemia and subsequent neurological injury. Hyperinsulinism is also the reason for hypoglycaemia in infants of diabetic mothers and in large for gestation-age (LGA) babies.

At-risk newborn babies
All newborn babies should be assessed for risk factors or potential causes for hypoglycaemia.[38] Babies born in good condition and who appear well at birth should have skin-to-skin contact and early feeding encouraged within the first hour of life. Skin-to-skin contact with the mother helps

maintain temperature and prevent cold stress. The risk factors and causes of hypoglycaemia can be classified into two groups: (1) those conditions associated with diminished hepatic glucose production and (2) conditions associated with hyperinsulinism.

Table 2 Causes of neonatal hypoglycaemia

Inadequate hepatic glucose production	Hyperinsulinism
Cold stress	Infant of diabetic mother
Congenital heart disease	Rhesus incompatibility
Cardiac failure	Beckwith-Weidemann syndrome
Inborn errors of metabolism: defective gluconeogenesis/glycogenolysis	Nesidioblastosis, islet cell adenoma
IUGR	Adrenal insufficiency
Prematurity	Beta-sympathomimetic exposure
Perinatal stress/hypoxia	Exchange transfusion and high UAC
Sepsis	Iatrogenic

History and examination

➤ There are no pathognomonic symptoms or signs for hypoglycaemia in neonates. It is important to remember that symptoms or signs may be present at different blood glucose concentrations in different neonates and may not be present at all in some neonates even with very low levels.

➤ In approximate order of frequency the symptoms and signs that may occur are jitteriness or tremors, apathy, episodes of cyanosis, convulsions, intermittent apnoeic spells or tachypnoea, weak or high-pitched cry, limpness or lethargy, difficulty in feeding, and eye rolling. Episodes of sweating, sudden pallor, hypothermia, and cardiac arrest and failure may occur.

➤ There is usually a clustering of episodic symptoms. These symptoms and signs can be a manifestation of various conditions, therefore it is very important to measure serum glucose levels and to determine if symptoms disappear and the glucose concentration rises to normal levels after administration of sufficient feed or glucose.

Management

When to check the capillary glucose:

➤ Babies who are well with no risk factors for the development of hypoglycaemia and have fed within the first hour do not need routine glucose monitoring. These babies can be fed on demand as long as they remain well. Feeding on demand does not mean waiting for the baby to cry with hunger. Crying is a late indicator of hunger. In the first few days especially, babies who are breastfed should be fed every 2–3 hours, offering the breast whenever the baby shows early signs of hunger such as increased alertness, physical activity, mouthing or rooting.

➤ Infants at risk of developing hypoglycaemia should have their blood glucose routinely measured at 2 hours of life and thereafter every 3–6 hours pre-feed, irrespective of the mode of feeding.

➤ In large for gestational-age babies and infants of diabetic mothers, if feeds are well established and glucose >2.6 mmol/L, monitoring can be stopped after 12 hours of age as hypoglycaemia beyond this time is unlikely.

➤ Small for gestational-age and preterm babies can develop hypoglycaemia as late as the second day of life and therefore it is reasonable to check the glucose once or twice on the second day of life. If feeding is well established and glucose >2.6 mmol/L, then monitoring can be stopped at 36 hours of age.

Management of a low glucose (see Algorithm)
Baby born in poor condition

➤ A baby born in poor condition should have glucose checked at the earliest opportunity. If <2.6 mmol/L give a 2–3 ml/kg bolus of 10% dextrose, followed by maintenance fluids as appropriate in the neonatal unit.

Baby born in good condition

➤ Babies born in good condition should have skin-to-skin contact
with the mother and be fed within the first 30–60 minutes of age.
Early and exclusive breastfeeding meets the nutritional requirements
of healthy term babies and they do not develop symptomatic
hypoglycaemia simply as a result of underfeeding. All babies should
be assessed for presence of the risk factors or potential causes of
neonatal hypoglycaemia.

Glucose <1.8 mmol/L at 2 hours or <2.6 mmol/L at subsequent checks

➤ If baby is symptomatic with apathy, episodes of cyanosis,
convulsions, intermittent apnoeic spells or tachypnoea, a weak or
high-pitched cry, limpness or lethargy, difficulty in feeding, episodes
of sweating, sudden pallor, hypothermia, cardiac arrest or failure –
administer 2–3 ml/kg of 10% dextrose intravenously over 1 minute
followed immediately by maintenance fluids with 10% dextrose
and admit to the neonatal unit for further investigations and
management.

➤ If baby is asymptomatic, check whether baby has had a feed, and if
not fed, then feed the baby and recheck the glucose after one hour.

➤ If BM is <2.6 mmol/L after the feed or at subsequent checks and
baby remains asymptomatic, then the options are: if breastfeeding,
increase frequency of feeding or the mother may express and feed
the baby by bottle/cup or consider giving top up of formula feeds
by bottle or cup, if it is thought that breast milk supply is less
than optimal. For babies who are bottle feeding: ensure feeding is
adequate by comparing what the baby is taking to their feeding
requirements based on their postnatal age. The low glucose should
be confirmed by checking a venous blood sugar. Consider using
low birth weight formula as this has more calories than standard
formula.

➤ A baby who is not feeding well or having poor suck should be assessed by medical staff for sepsis, heart disease, congenital pneumonia, etc.

➤ If glucose is <2.6 mmol/L on more than two occasions then the baby needs to be evaluated by medical staff. Appropriate investigations may include lab glucose, full blood picture, cultures, C-reactive protein, serum electrolytes, group and Coombs and capillary or venous blood gas. Admission to the neonatal unit for intravenous dextrose infusion must be strongly considered.

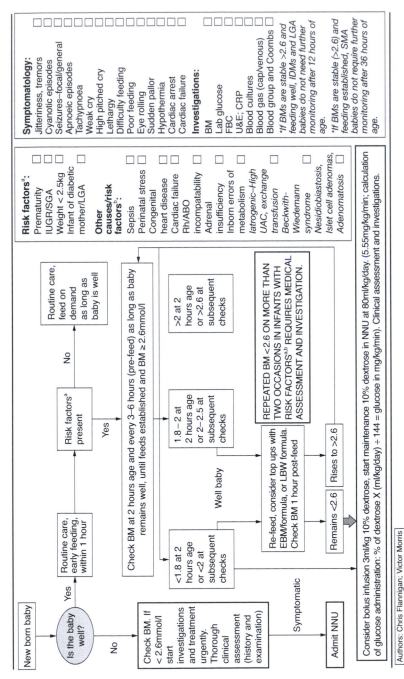

Figure 14 Algorithm for management of neonatal hypoglycaemia

Poor feeding

It is not uncommon for infants to have difficulty establishing feeding over the first few days of life. A newborn infant will often vomit over the first few days. Babies who are breastfed can have additional problems as learning the technique can take a little longer than bottle feeding for both mother and baby, and there can also be issues with poor supply of breast milk.

It is important that you are able to provide an accurate assessment of how feeding is going, exclude medical causes of poor feeding and provide useful advice on how to manage an infant who is feeding poorly.

History and examination

Enquire about the antenatal and perinatal history as to whether there are any clues about why the baby may be feeding poorly (for example was the baby preterm, was there polyhydramnios which can be associated with an upper gastrointestinal atresia, were there any risk factors for hypoxic-ischaemic encephalopathy at birth – low cord pH or prolonged resuscitation) and enquire about risk factors for sepsis.

For a bottle-fed baby enquire about how much the infant is taking per feed and how often the baby is feeding. Examine the feeding chart if available. Compare this to the baby's fluid requirements below.

Table 3 Typical neonatal fluid requirement depending on day of life

Day of life	Fluid requirements per 24-hour period
1	60 ml per kilogram
2	80 ml per kilogram
3	100 ml per kilogram
4	120 ml per kilogram
5	135 ml per kilogram
≥6	150 ml per kilogram

➤ Enquire about what the actual problem with the feeding is, e.g. not keen to take the feed, has difficulty sucking, becomes tired during the feed or vomiting post-feed.

➤ For a breastfed baby enquire about whether the mother/midwife is happy with the feeding technique and her supply of breast milk.

➤ Perform a full systemic examination of the infant but in particular look for problems that could explain the poor feeding, e.g. sepsis, respiratory distress, heart failure, blocked nasal passages, neurological problems or abnormality of the palate.

➤ Assess for signs of dehydration, e.g. dry mucous membranes, sunken anterior fontanelle and lethargy.

Management

➤ Check the capillary blood sugar in all babies with poor feeding, check the urea and electrolytes if there is evidence of dehydration and have a low threshold for performing a limited septic screen/ starting antibiotics if there are risk factors or signs of possible sepsis.

➤ Ask an experienced midwife to assess the feeding and offer advice on technique.

➤ For bottlefed babies advise the mother of the feeding requirements depending on the infant's day of life. Divide this 24-hour total by eight and ask her to feed the baby this volume every 3 hours and ask her to keep a feeding chart. Different shapes and sizes of teats should be tried.

➤ For breastfed babies ask the midwife to assess the technique and check the supply of breast milk by asking the mother to express at the time the next feed is due to see what volume she would have given the baby. If the amount of milk that the mother is able to express is below the infant's recommended requirements the infant should be offered a top-up of expressed breast milk/formula milk after the breastfeed. Provide encouragement for the mother to continue with the breastfeedings, explaining that the top-ups are only a temporary measure until her milk 'comes in'.

➤ Babies with feeding difficulties will require regular paediatric assessment on the postnatal ward, with particular attention paid to the baby's feeding record, capillary blood sugars and hydration status. If the baby is running into problems with any of the above, consider admission to the neonatal unit for tube feeds or intravenous fluids +/- further investigation.

Weight loss >10%

Over the first weeks of life it is normal for the newborn infant to fall below their birth weight for a number of reasons. First, they have moved from an environment where the placenta provides a constant supply of nutrients to one where they have to expand energy and take feeds for themselves. Also over the first few days milk intake is often suboptimal as feeding is established. For these reasons it is normal for a baby to lose up to 10% of their birth weight over the first week, which they should regain by around 10–14 days of age. If a baby has lost greater than 10% of their birth weight, a careful search for a cause should be made.

History and examination

➤ Feeding difficulty (e.g. poor supply of breast milk or not feeding adequate volumes of milk) is by far the most common cause. See the section of feeding problems for further information on important points to cover on history and examination.

➤ Enquire about any medical problems since birth. Any illness could help explain the weight loss. An unwell baby will often consume less calories than normal despite having a higher energy expenditure.

➤ If there is no obvious reason for the weight loss, a detailed history and full systemic examination should be performed to try and identify a cause. Specific attention should be paid to signs of hydration, heart failure and sepsis.

Management

➤ Your management should be directed towards any specific medical problem that is identified.

➤ If the weight loss is felt to be due to poor feeding, manage as per the section on feeding problems.

➤ If no cause for the weight loss can be identified through history and examination, recheck the accuracy of the measurement and if correct ask for a senior review.

➤ If the baby appears dehydrated check the electrolytes, as dehydration combined with weight loss greater than 10% of birth weight is often associated with hypernatraemia.

➤ The baby should have a daily weight documented and daily paediatric review on the postnatal ward.

➤ The baby can be discharged once the weight is no longer falling and the paediatric and midwifery teams are happy with the feeding.

➤ Arrange for the community midwife to continue monitoring the weight at home.

➤ Support the parents as it can be stressful for them, especially new mothers.

Vomiting

Vomiting over the first few days of life is not uncommon. Many of these babies are described as 'mucousy' and the vomiting is attributed to swallowed mucus irritating the baby's stomach combined with the process of gastro-oesophageal reflux. However, this must be differentiated from pathological causes of vomiting in the newborn.

Pathological causes of vomiting in the newborn include obstruction of the gastrointestinal tract from either congenital anomalies such as atresia of the oesophagus, bowel or anus, Hirschsprung's disease, meconium illeus or volvulus. Vomiting is also common in the septic infant, and can rarely indicate a neurological or metabolic condition.

History and examination

➤ Examine the mother's notes for evidence of polyhydramnios during the pregnancy as this can be a marker of obstruction of the upper gastrointestinal tract.

➤ Ask about the presence of bile in the vomit. Vomit containing yellow gastric juices will often be described as bilious and you must differentiate this from true bilious vomiting which is lime green in colour. This should be done by preferably examining the vomit yourself or by careful history taking. True bilious vomiting represents an obstruction distal to the ampulla of Vater till proven otherwise.

➤ Take a detailed feeding history.

➤ Ask about whether the infant appears in pain, or if there is any abdominal distention, and enquire about bowel habit.

➤ Assess the infant for signs of dehydration or sepsis.

➤ Look for any dysmorphic features or congenital abnormalities that can often be associated with an upper gastrointestinal atresia (e.g. vertebral, cardiac and limb abnormalities or anal atresia).

➤ Examine the abdomen, making comment on any distention, tenderness or masses and note the quality and intensity of the bowel sounds. Examine the groin for hernias and ensure the anus is patent.

Management

➤ In most cases there will be no red flag symptoms (e.g. bilious vomiting, abdominal distention or pain) in an infant who is well hydrated and feeding well. An explanation of the vomiting and reassurance should be offered to the parents.

➤ Consider checking the capillary blood sugar if the vomiting is frequent or persistent or if the infant displays signs of hypoglycaemia.

➤ If there are any concerns regarding possible sepsis perform a septic screen and start antibiotics.

➤ If the infant appears dehydrated or has persistent vomiting check the electrolytes and ask for a senior opinion, as admission to the neonatal unit for intravenous fluids +/- further investigation may be required.

➤ If the vomiting is persistent and occurs shortly after feeds, an upper gastrointestinal atresia should be excluded by passing an orogastric tube and ordering a chest/abdominal radiograph. In an oesophageal atresia the orogastric tube can be seen coiling in the oesophagus, while in a duodenal atresia a double bubble sign is seen on the radiograph.

➤ If there is true bilious vomiting, or if the infant has signs of an acute abdomen/intestinal obstruction on clinical examination:
  — admit to the neonatal unit
  — keep nil by mouth
  — pass an orogastric tube
  — order an abdominal radiograph
  — start intravenous fluids
  — request a surgical opinion.

Jittery

A baby who is described as 'jittery' can be observed having tremulous movements, most commonly involving the limbs. These movements can be differentiated from seizure activity simply by holding onto the limbs during an episode. In a seizure the shaking will continue, while in a baby who is 'jittery' the tremulous movement will stop.

There is a wide range of reasons why a baby may be jittery, but hypoglycaemia and substance withdrawal are probably responsible for the majority of cases. Nicotine withdrawal is probably the most common substance used during the pregnancy that results in jittery babies, but other substances used during the pregnancy that can result in jittery babies include caffeine, alcohol, numerous illicit or prescribed drugs (e.g. benzodiazepines, opioids or selective serotonin reuptake inhibitors).

Other causes that must be thought about include temperature instability, sepsis, jaundice, electrolyte disturbances (particularly low calcium and magnesium), hyperthyroidism and polycythaemia.

History and examination

➤ Enquire about what exactly happens during these episodes and in particular differentiate jittery movements from seizure activity or benign neonatal myoclonus: does it stop if you hold onto the infant's limbs? Is it associated with any colour change? Is the infant alert during the episodes? Does it only occur while sleeping? How frequently is it occurring?

➤ Enquire about risk factors for jittery movements: how is the feeding going? Did the mother smoke, drink alcohol or excessive caffeine during the pregnancy? Was she using any drugs prescribed or illicit drugs during the pregnancy? Does the mother have any thyroid problems?

➤ If the infant is having tremulous movements when you are there, hold onto the limb to see if this terminates the movement.

➤ Check the temperature, look for evidence of jaundice and examine the infant for any evidence of sepsis (lethargy, prolonged capillary refill time, tachycardia).

Management

➤ All babies who are felt to be jittery should have capillary blood sugar checked for evidence of hypoglycaemia.

➤ Whether you perform any further tests will depend on if a likely cause can be identified from history and examination, and how persistent or severe the jitteriness is.

➤ In a baby with no obvious cause for persistent jittery movements, a useful screen includes a full blood picture, urea and electrolytes, calcium, magnesium, bilirubin, C-reactive protein, blood glucose and thyroid function test.

Not passed urine

An infant should be expected to pass urine within 24 hours of birth. It can often be difficult to be certain whether an infant has passed urine or not, as the infant will normally pass meconium a number of times during the first 24 hours, which may mask the passage of urine. The infant may also have passed urine at birth and it may not have been documented. When this is combined with poor feeding and dehydration it increases the likelihood that urine will not be observed in the first 24 hours.

The most serious condition to exclude, particularly in a boy, is posterior urethral valves. In this condition the infant will fail to pass urine or only manage to pass a poor stream of urine. Clues to this diagnosis include oligohydramnios, bilateral hydronephrosis on antenatal scan and a palpable bladder or renal mass on clinical examination. If this condition is suspected, a renal ultrasound and micturating cystourethrogram should be requested and referral to a paediatric urologist made as the condition will require urinary catheter placement pre-surgery.

History and Examination

➤ Examine the mother's notes to check the infant was passing urine well antenatally (e.g. normal amniotic fluid volume and that there was no renal abnormality on the anomaly scan).

➤ Enquire about the infant's feeding and the mother's supply of milk if breastfeeding.

➤ Examine the infant's hydration (mucous membranes and anterior fontanelle), examine the abdomen for any masses including a palpable bladder and examine the external genitalia for any abnormality.

Management

➤ For the well-hydrated infant with no abnormality on examination it is useful to place some cotton balls into the nappy to detect the passage of any urine.

➤ If the infant is showing signs of dehydration ensure the infant is meeting their feeding requirements by topping up after a breastfeed if necessary. Consider checking the infant's urea and electrolytes and admitting to the neonatal unit if the problem persists.

➤ If urine output is still poor, discuss the infant with your senior. The baby may need an ultrasound scan of the kidneys and renal tracts +/- a micturating cystourethrogram to exclude posterior urethral valves.

Bowels not opened

Normally infants will pass meconium within the first 24 hours of life. If an infant has not passed meconium after 48 hours an underlying cause must be sought. Causes include anal atresia, Hirschsprung's disease, meconium illeus (which is associated with cystic fibrosis) and a meconium plug.

History and examination

➤ Enquire about a family history of bowel disorders including Hirschsprung's and cystic fibrosis.

➤ Enquire about the infant's feeding and ask about vomiting, especially bilious vomiting.

➤ Ensure the child has a patent anus, examine the abdomen for any distention, tenderness or masses and comment on the presence and character of the bowel sounds.

Management

➤ Order a plain abdominal radiograph and consult with a senior colleague.

➤ If the infant has associated vomiting admit promptly to the neonatal unit, pass an orogastric tube, measure urea and electrolytes and start intravenous fluids.

➤ It is likely the child will need referral to the paediatric surgeons for further investigation and treatment.

➤ Depending on the underlying diagnosis, further investigation may be required (e.g. screening for cystic fibrosis with meconium illeus and investigation for other associated malformations in anal atresia).

Sticky eyes

This is relatively common in neonates, and in the majority of cases it represents a blocked tear duct rather than infection. For persistent conjunctivitis resistant to treatment, infection with *chlamydia* or *gonorrhoea* should be considered. *Gonorrhoea* conjunctivitis tends to present within the first 48 hours of life, while *chlamydia* conjunctivitis classically presents around a week of age.

History and examination

➤ Examine the mother's notes for any risk factors for infection (e.g. prolonged rupture of membranes or previous sexually transmitted infections such as *chlamydia* or *gonorrhoea*.

➤ Check the infant's observations and perform a full systemic examination of the baby.

➤ Examine the eye in detail (including pupillary reactions and fundoscopy) and ensure there is no evidence of periorbital cellulitis.

Management

➤ Regular cleaning with sterile water and cotton wool for 24 hours.

➤ If no improvement after 24 hours swab eyes and start chloramphenicol or fucidin eye ointment.

➤ The majority of cases will settle with this management. If not, infection with *chlamydia* or *gonorrhoea* should be considered and appropriate swabs taken for gram staining and culture.

➤ Assess regularly for any evidence of developing periorbital cellulitis that will require intravenous antibiotics.

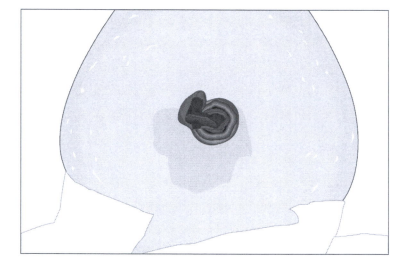

Figure 15 Omphalitis. Based on images courtesy of Newborn Services, Auckland City Hospital.[39]

Redness around umbilical cord

After birth when the umbilical cord has been cut, the remaining part of the cord is now dead tissue, which becomes necrotic and falls off around 5–7 days of age. The cord clamp can rub against the infant's skin, so it is not uncommon for there to be some mild erythema on the skin surrounding the umbilicus. This must be differentiated from an umbilical infection or omphalitis. Omphalitis is a serious condition in the neonate and if not treated quickly can result in sepsis, necrotising fasciitis and umbilical vessel phlebitis.

History and examination

➤ Ask whether the redness has spread from when it was first noticed.

➤ Examine the umbilicus for signs of infection. Probably the most important sign to look for is umbilical flare. This is spread of erythema from the raised skin next to the umbilical stump onto the flat surface of the abdomen, and it represents omphalitis. Other signs that the umbilicus may be infected include a foul smell or discharge from the umbilicus, peeling, blistering or induration of the skin and tenderness on palpation.

If you suspect the umbilicus is infected look for evidence of sepsis in the neonate, e.g. a history of poor feeding and lethargy, jaundice, pyrexia and signs of shock (tachycardia and prolonged capillary refill time).

Management

➤ In well babies with mild erythema and no evidence of omphalitis it is reasonable to remove the cord clamp and review the baby again in a few hours time. If the erythema is secondary to rubbing from the cord clamp it should improve over this time period.

➤ Mark the area of erythema with a ballpoint pen so you will know if it is spreading or not. Tell the mother/midwife not to wash it off!

➤ For suspected omphalitis insert an intravenous line and take blood for full blood picture, C-reactive protein, blood culture and swab the cord.

➤ Start the baby on appropriate intravenous antibiotics after obtaining cultures and swab, e.g. flucloxacillin and benzylpenicillin.

➤ Regular paediatric review and observations will be required on the postnatal wards in the well infant, who if at any stage displays signs of sepsis should be admitted to the neonatal unit without delay.

Pink staining on nappy

Urates are pink/orange crystals that are commonly found in the urine of newborn infants. They are a normal finding in a newborn and don't require any further investigation. They are more common when infants are dehydrated, but are often found in well-hydrated infants.

History and examination

➤ Ensure the nappy contains a pink/orange stain from where the urine has soaked into it and not blood.

➤ Examine baby to ensure no evidence of bleeding from nappy region or umbilical cord.

➤ Enquire about feeding and examine for signs of dehydration.

Management

➤ Parental reassurance.

Vaginal bleeding

Vaginal bleeding is a normal physiological process in the newborn female baby. In utero the infant is exposed to high levels of maternal oestrogens which stimulate the neonatal endometrium. It is the withdrawal of the oestrogen at birth that causes a white vaginal discharge often followed by bleeding.

History and examination

➤ Perform a full systemic examination of the neonate excluding bruising and bleeding from elsewhere.

➤ Examine the genitalia to ensure it is normal with no evidence of trauma.

Management

➤ Reassurance of the parents with an explanation of why this occurs is all that is required.

➤ Advise them that if the discharge becomes foul smelling they should seek a medical opinion.

Maternal thyroid disease

In the UK all neonates should be screened for congenital hypothyroidism by measuring the thyroid stimulating hormone on a Guthrie card. Provided the baby is asymptomatic and the maternal history is of isolated hypothyroidism (i.e. she was never hyperthyroid), no further investigation is required.

In maternal Graves disease, thyroid stimulating immunoglobulins can cross the placenta and cause neonatal thyrotoxicosis. Even in Graves disease neonatal thyrotoxicosis is rare, but as the mortality rate from neonatal thyrotoxicosis is around 12–20% the condition must be actively sought even in asymptomatic infants.[40]

History and Examination

➤ Even when there is a documented history of hypothyroidism, always ask the mother if she ever had hyperthyroidism. A woman who had Graves disease in the past, was treated and is now clinically hypothyroid or euthyroid can still have thyroid stimulating immunoglobulin in her blood that can cross the placenta.

➤ Enquire about the infant's feeding and level of alertness, and ask about sweating, tachypnoea, weight loss and diarrhoea.

➤ Examine the infant for signs of thyrotoxicosis, e.g. goitre, tachypnoea, tachycardia, sweating, jitteriness and irritability.

Management

➤ In an asymptomatic infant with an isolated history of maternal hypothyroidism, nothing more than the routine Guthrie test is required.

➤ For infants of mothers who were hyperthyroid at any stage it is useful to send cord blood for thyroid function tests.

➤ Explain the signs of hyperthyroidism to the parents and arrange for the baby to have thyroid function tests checked again between 10 and 14 days of age.

➤ If at any stage the infant displays signs of thyrotoxicosis check the thyroid function tests urgently and ask for a senior opinion. It is likely that the infant will require treatment in hospital.

Maternal hepatitis B

Mothers who are carriers for hepatitis B can pass the infection on to their infants around the time of birth. Therefore all babies whose mothers are known carriers for hepatitis B should be offered immunisation and in most cases hepatitis B immunoglobulin. If the mother is anti-HBe positive this reduces the risk of transmission to the infant and only the vaccine will be required.

Table 4 Treatment required according to hepatitis B status of mother[41]

	Hepatitis B immunisation	Hepatitis B immunoglobulin
Mother is HBsAg Positive and HBeAg positive	Yes	Yes
Mother is HBsAg Positive, HBeAg negative and anti-HBe negative	Yes	Yes
Mother is HBsAg Positive, e-markers not determined	Yes	Yes
Mother had acute hepatitis during pregnancy	Yes	Yes
Mother is HBsAg Positive and anti-HBe positive	Yes	No

History and examination

➤ Check the mother's notes for her hepatitis B serology to help decide whether immunoglobulin will also be required.

➤ Also look for evidence of any other maternal infective diseases that may require further action in the neonate, e.g. HIV or *chlamydia*.

Management

➤ Obtain informed consent from the mother for vaccination +/- immunoglobulin and aim to administer the vaccination shortly after birth.

➤ 10 micrograms of hepatitis B vaccination (Energix) should be administered intramuscularly into the anterolateral thigh.

➤ If hepatitis B immunoglobulin is required administer 200 international units intramuscularly into the opposite anterolateral thigh.

➤ Document in the baby's notes, medicine chart and 'red book'.

➤ Arrange follow-up according to local practice as further doses of vaccine will be required at one month and two months, with a booster being given at 12 months of age.

BCG vaccination

In the UK the BCG vaccination is no longer given routinely to all children at school. Instead, since 2005, all high-risk newborns should be vaccinated.

History and examination

You should carry out a risk factor assessment in all infants on routine discharge examination to assess the need for a BCG vaccination. If any of the following risk factors are present the infant should be offered the vaccination:[42]

1 Infants whose parents or grandparents were born in a high-risk country. A country is regarded as high risk if it has an incidence of TB greater than 40/100 000. (Countries' incidents of TB can be checked at the Health Protection Agencies website.)[43]

2 Infants who will spend more than one month living in a high-risk country.

3 If there is anyone in the household who had or is suspected of having TB in the last five years.

Management

➤ Check that the mother is HIV negative. BCG should not be given at birth to infants of HIV-positive mothers.

➤ Obtain written informed consent for the BCG vaccination.

➤ Obtain the help of an assistant to hold the baby's arm still during the procedure.

➤ Withdraw 0.05 ml of the BCG vaccination in a 1 ml syringe and change to a clean small needle.

➤ Clean lateral surface of the left upper arm. The injection site is at the lower insertion of the deltoid muscle.

➤ Stretch the skin over the injection site so that it is taut, and insert the needle with the bevel pointing upwards parallel to the skin as superficially as possible (this is an intradermal injection, not subcutaneous).

➤ Inject the vaccine: you should see a small white bleb forming if you have done the procedure correctly. Record whether a bleb was raised or not.

➤ Remember to record the batch number on the vaccination consent form and to record that you have given the vaccination in the parent-held child record 'red book'.

Vitamin K

Prevention of vitamin K deficiency bleeding (VKDB) of the newborn (previously known as haemorrhagic disease of the newborn) is now routine policy throughout the UK. While both oral and parenteral vitamin K offer adequate protection against early VKDB, there is increasing evidence that parenteral vitamin K is more effective than oral vitamin K in preventing late VKDB,[44] and as a result many units are now offering intramuscular vitamin K as standard. As breast milk has less vitamin K than formula milk, breastfed infants are at higher risk of VKDB (particularly late onset).

In the past there have been some concerns about the possible association between parenteral vitamin K and childhood cancer. These concerns have not been sustained[44] and parents should be reassured.

Management

➤ Obtain informed consent from the parents for the administration of intramuscular vitamin K.

➤ For a term infant administer 1 mg of phytomenadione intramuscularly into the anterolateral thigh.

➤ For preterm infants administer 400 micrograms per kilogram (up to a maximum dose of 1 mg)[45] of phytomenadione intramuscularly into the anterolateral thigh.

➤ Parents refusing intramuscular vitamin K should be advised that it is the most effective way to prevent VKDB. Oral vitamin K should be offered as an alternative.

➤ The dosing regime for oral vitamin K involves 2 mg of Konakion MM™ being given orally at birth and a second dose within a week of birth for all infants. A third dose is required at one month of age for all breastfed infants.[44]

➤ If parents refuse vitamin K make clear notes documenting your discussion with them, in particular that you have explained the risk and complications of VKDB including intracranial bleeding.

Notes

1 Rudolph MA, Kamei RK. *Rudolph's Fundamentals of Pediatrics*. 2002. McGraw-Hill Medical: p. 667.

2 Jones R, Hunt A. Current management of clubfoot (congenital talipes equinovarus). *BMJ*. 2010; **7741**: 308–12. www.bmj.com/cgi/content/extract/340/feb02_1/c355

3 Rennie JM. Examining the normal neonate. *Current Paediatrics*. 2004; **14**: 361–65. www.journals.elsevierhealth.com/periodicals/ycuoe/article/PIIS0957583904000442/abstract

4 Kriss VM, Desai NS. Occult spinal dysraphism in neonates: assessment of high-risk cutaneous stigmata on sonography. *AJR Am J Roentgenol*. 1998; **171**: 1687–92. www.ajronlineorg/cgi/content/abstract/171/6/1687?ijkey=0f3b2d476bcd812e9808e9996f1b62ed49c38a29&keytype2=tf_ipsecsha

5 Arora R, Pryce R. Is ultrasound required to rule out renal malformations in babies with isolated preauricular tags? *Arch Dis Child*. 2004; **89**: 492–93. http://adc.bmj.com/cgi/content/full/89/5/492

6 Newborn Services, Auckland City Hospital. Ear abnormalities. www.adhb.govt.nz/newborn/TeachingResources/Dermatology/EarAnomalies.htm

7 Laroia N. Birth trauma. *Emedicine*. 2008. http://emedicine.medscape.com/article/980112-overview

8 National Institute for Health and Clinical Excellence. Division of ankyloglossia for breastfeeding. NICE. 2005. www.nice.org.uk/nicemedia/pdf/ip/IPG149guidance.pdf

9 Tolarova M. Cleft lip and palate. *Emedicine*. 2009. http://emedicine.medscape.com/article/995535-overview

10 Cleft Lip & Palate Association (CLAPA). www.clapa.com

11 Brachial plexus palsies: long-term followup. *Arch Dis Child Educ Pract Ed*. 2007; **92**: 96. http://ep.bmj.com/content/92/3/ep96.full

12 Rao P, Seib P. Coarctation of the aorta. *Emedicine*. 2009. http://emedicine.medscape.com/article/895502-overview

13 Crossland D, Furness J, Abu-Harb M, *et al*. Variability of four limb blood pressure in normal neonates. *Arch Dis Child Fetal Neonatal Ed*. 2004; **89**: 325–27. http://fn.bmjjournals.com/content/89/4/F325.full

14 Bauchner H. Developmental dysplasia of the hip (DDH): an evolving science. *Arch Dis Child.* 2000; **83**: 202. http://adc.bmj.com/content/83/3/202.full

15 Committee on Quality Improvement, American Academy of Pediatrics. Clinical practice guidelines: early detection of developmental dysplasia of the hip. *Pediatrics.* 2000; **105**: 896–905. http://pediatrics.aappublications. org/cgi/content/full/105/4/896?ijkey=e8b2c56354a83c2619074a71618f4f a7bb18f7ea

16 Beall M, Ross M. Umbilical cord complications. *Emedicine.* 2009. http:// emedicine.medscape.com/article/262470-overview

17 Srinivasan R, Arora R. Do well infants born with an isolated single umbilical artery need investigation? *Arch Dis Child.* 2005; **90**: 100–01. http://adc.bmj.com/content/90/1/100.full?sid=a6f9a966-41c8-441f-8b3f-db3a612bdc3d

18 Newborn Services, Auckland City Hospital. Other lesions. www.adhb.govt. nz/newborn/TeachingResources/Dermatology/OtherLesions htm

19 European Association of Urology, European Society for Paediatric Urology. *Guidelines on Paediatric Urology.* 2009. www.guideline.gov/summary/ summary.aspx?doc_id=12594

20 Hatch J, DPM, FACFAS. Foot & Ankle Centre of Northern Colorado PC.

21 Williams H. Spinal sinuses, dimples, pits and patches: what lies beneath? *Arch Dis Child Educ Pract Ed.* 2006; **91**: 75–80. http://ep.bmj.com/cgi/ content/full/91/3/ep75

22 Newborn Services, Auckland City Hospital. Back and scalp lesions. www. adhb.govt.nz/newborn/TeachingResources/Dermatology/BackLesions.htm

23 Newborn Services, Auckland City Hospital. Vascular lesions. www.adhb. govt.nz/newborn/TeachingResources/Dermatology/VascularLesions.htm

24 Beute T, Gibbs N, Huff R, *et al.* Erythema toxicum neonatorum. *Emedicine.* 2009. http://emedicine.medscape.com/article/1110731-overview

25 Sorrell J, Laumann A. Transient neonatal pustular melanosis. *Emedicine.* 2009. http://emedicine.medscape.com/article/1112258-overview

26 Silverman R. Neonatal pustular melanosis. *Emedicine.* 2009. http:// emedicine.medscape.com/article/909753-overview

27 Newborn Services, Auckland City Hospital. Benign lesions. www.adhb. govt.nz/newborn/TeachingResources/Dermatology/BenignLesions.htm

28 Toth B, Becker A, Seelbach-Gobel B. Oxygen saturations in healthy newborn infants immediately after birth measured by pulse oximetry. *Arch Gynecol Obstet.* 2002; **266**: 105–07. www.springerlink.com/content/ xc0fl69m0byek2re/fulltext.pdf?page=1

29 Anderson-Berry A, Bellig L, Ohning B. Neonatal sepsis. *Emedicine*. 2008. http://emedicine.medscape.com/article/978352overview

30 Flannigan C, Hogan M. Prolonged rupture of membranes in term infants: should all babies be screened? *Clinical Audit*. 2010; **2**: 1–6. http://www.dovepress.com/prolonged-rupture-of-membranes-in-term-infants-should-all-babies-be-sc-peer-reviewed-article-CA

31 National Institute for Health and Clinical Excellence. CG55 Intrapartum care. RCOG Press; 2007. www.nice.org.uk/nicemedia/pdf/CG55FullGuideline.pdf

32 American Academy of Pediatrics (AAP) Guidelines. Management of hyperbilirubinemia in the newborn infant 35 or more weeks of gestation. 2004. http://aappolicy.aappublications.org/cgi/content/full/pediatrics;114/1/297

33 Swenne I, Ewald U, Gustafsson J, *et al*. Inter-relationship between serum concentrations of glucose, glucagon and insulin during first two days of life in healthy newborns. *Acta Paediatr*. 1994; **83**: 915–19. www3.interscience.wiley.com/journal/119971560/abstract?CRETRY=1&SRETRY=0

34 World Health Organization. Neonatal hypoglycaemia: a review of literature. 1997. WHO/CHD/97_1. http://whqlibdoc.who.int/hq/1997 WHO_CHD_97.1.pdf

35 Cornblath M, Hawdon J, Williams A, *et al*. Controversies regarding definition of neonatal hypoglycaemia: suggested operational threshold. *Pediatrics*. 2000; **105**: 1141–45. http://pediatrics.aappublications.org/cgi/content/abstract/105/5/1141

36 Sunehag A, Haymond M. Glucose extremes in newborn infants. *Clin Perinatol*. 2002; **29**: 245–60. www.mdconsult.com/das/article/body/177761368-2/jorg=journal&source=&sp=12597002&sid=0/N/290750/1.html?issn=00955108

37 Jerome Y, Yager MD. Hypoglycaemic injury to the immature brain. *Clinics in Perinatology*. 2002; **29**: 651–74.

38 de Lonlay P, Giurgea I, Touati G, Saudubray J-M. Neonatal hypoglycaemia: aetiologies. *Semin Neonato*. 2004; **9**: 49–58. www.siem.ufrgs.br/artigos/hipoglicemianeonatal.pdf

39 Newborn Services, Auckland City Hospital. Infective lesions. www.adhb.govt.nz/newborn/TeachingResources/Dermatology/InfectiveLesions.htm

40 Ogilvy-Stuart A. Neonatal thyroid disorders. *Arch Dis Child Fetal Neonatal Ed*. 2002; **87**: 165–71. http://fn.bmj.com/content/87/3/F165.full?sid=626f6d71-509b-4d89-9e33-b73187b738cb

41 Department of Health. Hepatitis B: immunisation against infectious diseases. 'The Green Book'. 2006. Department of Health; **18**: 161–84.

www.dh.gov.uk/dr_consum_dh/groups/dh_digitalassets/@dh/@en/ documents/digitalasset/dh_108820.pdf

42 Department of Health. Tuberculosis: immunisation against infectious diseases. 'The Green Book'. 2006; **32**: 391–408. www.dh.gov.uk/dr_consum_ dh/groups/dh_digitalassets/@dh/@en/documents/digitalasset/dh_108824. pdf

43 Health Protection Agency. WHO estimates of tuberculosis incidence by country. 2007. www.hpa.org.uk/web/HPAweb&HPAwebStandard/HPA web_C/1195733758290

44 American Academy of Pediatrics. Controversies concerning vitamin K and the newborn. *Pediatrics*. 2003; **112**: 191–92. http://aappolicy.aappublications. org/cgi/reprint/pediatrics;112/1/191.pdf

45 Paediatric Formulary Committee. *BNF for Children 2009*. London: BMJ Publishing Group, RPS Publishing and RCPCH Publications; 2009.

Further reading

Cleft Lip & Palate Association (CLAPA). www.clapa.com

Department of Health. Immunisation against infectious diseases. 'The Green Book'. 2006. www.dh.gov.uk/en/Publichealth/Healthprotection/Immunisation/Greenbook/DH_4097254

National Institute for Health and Clinical Excellence. CG037 Routine postnatal care of women and their babies. NICE. 2007. www.nice.org.uk/nicemedia/pdf/CG037fullguideline.pdf

Newborn Emergency Transport Service (Victoria). *Neonatal Handbook*. www.netsvic.org.au/nets/handbook/index.cfm?tabnav=all

Newborn Services, Auckland City Hospital. *Clinical Guidelines Index*. www.adhb.govt.nz/newborn/Guidelines.htm

Newborn Services, Auckland City Hospital. www.adhb.govt.nz/newborn/TeachingResources/Dermatology/Dermatology.htm

Stanford School of Medicine, Newborn Nursery, Photo Gallery Index. http://newborns.stanford.edu/PhotoGallery/GalleryIndex.html

DVD contents

1. **The Newborn Check:** demonstration by a neonatologist of how to perform a routine newborn discharge examination.
2. **Common Postnatal Problems – Part One:** advises on dealing with the 'big three' problems: the hips, the heart and the eyes.
3. **Common Postnatal Problems – Part Two:** addresses the management of birth trauma, neonatal conjunctivitis, umbilical infections, hydroceles, undescended testes and sacral dimples.
4. **Common Postnatal Problems – Part Three:** includes tips for treating small for gestational age babies, large for gestational age babies, jittery babies, talipes and feeding problems.
5. **Hypoglycaemia:** focuses on prevention of and screening for hypoglycaemia, and covers the different treatment options available.
6. **Hydronephrosis:** covers the potential causes of antenatal hydronephrosis and offers advice on the postnatal investigation and management.
7. **Jaundice:** provides a stepwise approach to the investigation and management of neonatal jaundice by dividing the condition into jaundice which is 'too early' (first 24 hours of life), 'too high' (hyperbilirubinaemia) or 'too long; (prolonged jaundice).

Index

Note: page numbers in **bold** refer to figures and tables.

ABC approach 57–8
abdomen, in newborn check 3
abdominal examination 32–3, 67, 82–3, 86
acetabulum 4, 28
acidosis 51, 66
alcohol 84; *see also* fetal alcohol syndrome
amblyopia 12, 47
anaemia 64, 66
antenatal anomaly scan 56, 58
anterior fontanelle
    bulging 61
    and hydration 86
    sunken 67, 78
antibiotics
    and breast swelling 23
    and feeding 78
    and omphalitis 92
    prophylactic 59, 62
    and sepsis 61–3
    and tachycardia 56
    and vomiting 83
antibodies 45, 64–6
atresia 77, 82–3, 88

Barlow's manoeuvre 4, 28–9
BCG vaccination 99–100
bile 82
bilirubin 64–9, 85

birthmarks 47
blood cultures
    and breast swelling 23
    and sepsis 56, 60–2
blood glucose 70, 72–3, 85
blood picture 8, 23, 45, 56, 59, 68–9, 75, 85, 92
blood pressures, four limb 26
blood tests 62, 68
bottle feeding 74, 77–8
bowel disorders 88
bradycardia 58
breast milk, supply of 74, 77–8, 80, 86
breast swelling 23
breastfeeding
    and hypoglycaemia 73–4
    and jaundice 64, 67
    problems with 16
breech presentation 28
bruising 8, 15, 45, 64, 66–7, 94

caesarean section 51, 54
caffeine 84
capillary blood sugar 78–9, 83, 85
capillary refill time 25, 52, 55–8, 60–1, 67
caput succedaneum 2, 7–8
cardiac arrest 72, 74
cardiac arrhythmias 56, 58
cardiac examination, newborn 2

cardiovascular system (CVS), examination 24, 26
cataracts 11–12
cavernous haemangioma, *see* strawberry naevus
cephalhaematoma 2, 7–8, 64, 66
cerebral palsy 65
chignon 7
chlamydia 89, 97
chorioamnionitis 59, 61
clavicles 3, 8, 20–1
cleft lip and palate 17, 18–19
congenital adrenal hyperplasia 35, 39
conjunctivitis 89
Coombs test 64–8, 75–6
crepitus 3, 20
CRP (C-reactive protein)
    and breast swelling 23
    and hypoglycaemia 75
    and jittery babies 85
    and sepsis 56, 59–60, 69
CRT, *see* capillary refill time
cryptorchidism 39
cyanosis 24–6, 54–5, 72, 74
cystic fibrosis 88

DDH (developmental dysplasia of the hip) 28–9
dehydration 56, 67–8, 78, 81–3, 86–7, 93
diabetic mothers 52, 66, 71, 73
double bubble sign 83
drugs 84

ECG, *see* electrocardiogram
echocardiography 24, 27
electrocardiogram 25, 27, 56, 58
electrolytes 75, 78, 81, 83–5, 87–8
elliptocytosis 65–6
Erb's palsy 20–1
erythema 23, 61, 91

erythema toxicum 48–9, **48**
eyes
    in newborn check 4
    sticky 89

facial nerve palsy 8, 15
feeding, establishing 77–9
femoral pulses 2, 24–7, 52, 55
fetal alcohol syndrome 22
forceps 8, 15, 45
foreskin 3, 39

GBS (group B streptococcus) 59–62
genitalia
    ambiguous 35, 39
    in newborn check 3
glucose
    capillary 73
    metabolism of 70–1
glucose-6-phosphate dehydrogenase (G6PD) 66
glycogen-6-phosphatase 71
gonorrhoea 89
Graves disease 95
groin swelling 34
group B streptococcus (GBS) 59–62
Guthrie test 95

Haberman feeder 17
haemolysis 65–8
haemorrhage
    intracranial 15
    subaponeurotic 7–9
hearing tests 14
heart block 58
heart disease
    congenital 24, 26, 55
    cyanotic 54
heart failure 25, 51–2, 78, 80

heart murmurs 24–5, 55
heart rate, in newborn check 2
hepatic glycogenolysis 71
hepatitis B 97–8, **97**
hepatomegaly 25, 52
hepatosplenomegaly 45, 67
hernias
    diaphragmatic 51–2
    inguinal 34, 37
    umbilical **31**, 32
    and vomiting 83
hips
    developmental dysplasia of,
      see DDH
    dislocation of 3–4, 28
Hirschsprung's disease 82, 88
HIV 97, 99
hydroceles **36**, 37
hydronephrosis 86
hyperbilirubinaemia 65–7
hyperglycaemia 70
hyperinsulinism 71–2
hyperthyroidism 84, 95
hypoglycaemia 70–5, 83–5
    algorithm for management of
    76
    causes of **72**
hypoplasia, pulmonary 52
hypospadias **38**, 39
hypothermia 58, 72, 74
hypothyroidism 32, 58, 95
hypoxic-ischaemic encephalopathy
  58, 77

immunoglobulin 95, 97–8
infections, congenital 65
intersex 39

jaundice
    and bruising 45
    causes of 64–5

examination for 66–7
and jittery babies 84–5
management of 67–9
and scalp swelling 8
jittery babies 84–5, 95

LGA (large for gestation age) 71, 73
lumbosacral lipomas 43–4

mastitis 23
meconium 3, 86, 88
meconium aspiration syndrome 51–3
meconium stained liquor 52, 54
membranes, prolonged rupture of
  (PROM) 59–62, 89
micturating cystourethrogram 30, 86–7
Moro reflex 4, 20–1
mucous membranes 67, 78, 86
myoclonus 84

nasal flaring 3, 51
neonatal fluid requirement **77**
neonatal intensive care unit (NICU) 25
newborn examination 1–5

occult spinal dysraphism 43, 47
oedema 2, 7
oligohydramnios 52, 86
omphalitis 90, 91–2
Ortolani's manoeuvre 3–4, 28–9
oxygen saturations 26, 52–6, 58

patent ductus arteriosus (PDA) 26, 54
penis 39
periorbital cellulitis 89
peripheries, cold 26, 52
phototherapy 66–9
pneumonia, congenital 51–4, 75
pneumothorax 51–4
polycythaemia 51, 66, 84
polyhydramnios 77, 82

port wine stain 46–7, **46**

positive pressure ventilation 51–2

precordium 24

processus vaginalis 34, 37

PROM, *see* membranes, prolonged
  rupture of

pyrexia 56, 59–60, 91

radiography 20–1, 25, 27, 53, 83

rashes **48**, 49–50

recti, divarication of 33

'red book' 5, 35, 98, 100

red reflex 4, **10**, 11–12

renal malformations 30

renal masses 86

respiratory distress
  and cyanosis 54
  and feeding 78
  management of 52–3
  in newborn check 3
  signs of 51–2, 54–5

respiratory distress syndrome (RDS)
  51–2, 54

respiratory rate, in newborn check 2

resuscitation 52, 54, 58
  fluid 9
  prolonged 77

Rhesus disease 64–5

sacral dimple 42–3, **42**

salmon patches 46–7, **46**

scalp swelling 7–9

scrotal swelling 37

sepsis
  and feeding 78
  and hypoglycaemia 75
  and infected umbilicus 91–2
  and jaundice 66–7, 69
  and jittery babies 84–5
  management of 61–2
  and omphalitis 91

and rashes 49

and respiratory distress 51

risk factors for 59–60

signs of 62–3

and tachycardia 56

and vomiting 82–3

and weight loss 80

shoulder dystocia 8, 20–1

simple dimple 4, 43

single palmar creases 22

skin tags 43–4
  preauricular 2, **13**, **14**

skin-to-skin contact 71, 74

spherocytosis 65

spine, in newborn check 4

Staphylococcus aureus 23

strawberry naevus 46–7, **46**

Sturge–Weber syndrome 47

substance withdrawal 56, 84

suture lines 2, 7–8

SVT (supraventricular tachycardia)
  56–7

sweating 26, 52, 72, 74, 95

systemic lupus erythematosus (SLE)
  58

tachycardia
  and heart murmurs 25
  management of 56–7
  and respiratory distress 52
  and scalp swelling 8
  and sepsis 67
  and subaponeurotic haemorrhage 8
  supraventricular, *see* SVT
  and thyrotoxicosis 95

tachypnoea
  and absent femorals 26
  and heart murmur 25
  transient, *see* TTN

talipes 4, 28, 40, 41

testes 3, 35, 37, 39

thyrotoxicosis 56, 95–6
tongue-tie 16
transient pustular melanosis
   48, 48–9
trisomy 21 22, 32
TTN (transient tachypnoea of the
   newborn) 51–2, 54
tuberculosis 99

ultrasound
   and heart disease 24, 55
   of hips 29
   renal 14, 30, 86–7
   spinal 44
umbilical cord 30, 61, 91–3

umbilical hernia, *see* hernias, umbilical
urates 93
urethral meatus 38, 39
urine 3, 39, 63, 86–7, 93

vaginal bleeding 94
vaginal discharge 3, 94
ventouse 7–8, 45
vesicoureteral reflux 30
vitamin K 8, 45
vitamin K deficiency bleeding
   (VKDB) 101
vomiting 77, 82–3, 88

weight loss 80–1, 95